Minimally Invasive Heart Surgery

Minimally Invasive Heart Surgery

Guest Editor
Manuel Wilbring

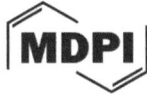 Basel • Beijing • Wuhan • Barcelona • Belgrade • Novi Sad • Cluj • Manchester

Guest Editor
Manuel Wilbring
Department of Cardiac Surgery
University Heart Center Dresden
Dresden
Germany

Editorial Office
MDPI AG
Grosspeteranlage 5
4052 Basel, Switzerland

This is a reprint of the Special Issue, published open access by the journal *Journal of Clinical Medicine* (ISSN 2077-0383), freely accessible at: www.mdpi.com/journal/jcm/special_issues/N926K6065N.

For citation purposes, cite each article independently as indicated on the article page online and using the guide below:

Lastname, A.A.; Lastname, B.B. Article Title. *Journal Name* **Year**, *Volume Number*, Page Range.

ISBN 978-3-7258-3436-5 (Hbk)
ISBN 978-3-7258-3435-8 (PDF)
https://doi.org/10.3390/books978-3-7258-3435-8

© 2025 by the authors. Articles in this book are Open Access and distributed under the Creative Commons Attribution (CC BY) license. The book as a whole is distributed by MDPI under the terms and conditions of the Creative Commons Attribution-NonCommercial-NoDerivs (CC BY-NC-ND) license (https://creativecommons.org/licenses/by-nc-nd/4.0/).

Contents

About the Editor vii

Manuel Wilbring
Advancing Minimally Invasive Cardiac Surgery—Let's Take a Look into the Future
Reprinted from: *J. Clin. Med.* **2025**, *14*, 904, https://doi.org/10.3390/jcm14030904 1

Ali Taghizadeh-Waghefi, Asen Petrov, Sebastian Arzt, Konstantin Alexiou, Klaus Matschke and Utz Kappert et al.
Minimally Invasive Aortic Valve Replacement for High-Risk Populations: Transaxillary Access Enhances Survival in Patients with Obesity
Reprinted from: *J. Clin. Med.* **2024**, *13*, 6529, https://doi.org/10.3390/jcm13216529 5

Sadeq Ali-Hasan-Al-Saegh, Florian Helms, Khalil Aburahma, Sho Takemoto, Nunzio Davide De Manna and Lukman Amanov et al.
Can Obesity Serve as a Barrier to Minimally Invasive Mitral Valve Surgery? Overcoming the Limitations—A Multivariate Logistic Regression Analysis
Reprinted from: *J. Clin. Med.* **2024**, *13*, 6355, https://doi.org/10.3390/jcm13216355 20

Jawad Salman, Maximilian Franz, Khalil Aburahma, Nunzio Davide de Manna, Saleh Tavil and Sadeq Ali-Hasan-Al-Saegh et al.
Hypothermic Ventricular Fibrillation in Redo Minimally Invasive Mitral Valve Surgery: A Promising Solution for a Surgical Challenge
Reprinted from: *J. Clin. Med.* **2024**, *13*, 4269, https://doi.org/10.3390/jcm13144269 34

Maximilian Franz, Khalil Aburahma, Fabio Ius, Sadeq Ali-Hasan-Al-Saegh, Dietmar Boethig and Nora Hertel et al.
Minimally Invasive Surgery through Right Mini-Thoracotomy for Mitral Valve Infective Endocarditis: Contraindicated or Safely Possible?
Reprinted from: *J. Clin. Med.* **2024**, *13*, 4182, https://doi.org/10.3390/jcm13144182 43

Florian Piekarski, Marc Rohner, Nadejda Monsefi, Farhad Bakhtiary and Markus Velten
Anesthesia for Minimal Invasive Cardiac Surgery: The Bonn Heart Center Protocol
Reprinted from: *J. Clin. Med.* **2024**, *13*, 3939, https://doi.org/10.3390/jcm13133939 50

Alexander Weymann, Lukman Amanov, Eleftherios Beltsios, Arian Arjomandi Rad, Marcin Szczechowicz and Ali Saad Merzah et al.
Minimally Invasive Direct Coronary Artery Bypass Grafting: Sixteen Years of Single-Center Experience
Reprinted from: *J. Clin. Med.* **2024**, *13*, 3338, https://doi.org/10.3390/jcm13113338 62

Florian Helms, Ezin Deniz, Heike Krüger, Alina Zubarevich, Jan Dieter Schmitto and Reza Poyanmehr et al.
Minimally Invasive Approach for Replacement of the Ascending Aorta towards the Proximal Aortic Arch
Reprinted from: *J. Clin. Med.* **2024**, *13*, 3274, https://doi.org/10.3390/jcm13113274 72

Martín Moscoso-Ludueña, Maximilian Vondran, Marc Irqsusi, Holger Nef, Ardawan J. Rastan and Tamer Ghazy
Combined Minimally Invasive Mitral Valve Surgery and Percutaneous Coronary Intervention: A Hybrid Concept for Patients with Mitral Valve and Coronary Pathologies
Reprinted from: *J. Clin. Med.* **2023**, *12*, 5553, https://doi.org/10.3390/jcm12175553 80

Ali Taghizadeh-Waghefi, Asen Petrov, Philipp Jatzke, Manuel Wilbring, Utz Kappert and Klaus Matschke et al.
Minimally Invasive Isolated Aortic Valve Replacement in a Potential TAVI Cohort of Patients Aged ⩾ 75 Years: A Propensity-Matched Analysis
Reprinted from: *J. Clin. Med.* **2023**, *12*, 4963, https://doi.org/10.3390/jcm12154963 . . . . **90**

Jade Claessens, Pieter Goris, Alaaddin Yilmaz, Silke Van Genechten, Marithé Claes and Loren Packlé et al.
Patient-Centred Outcomes after Totally Endoscopic Cardiac Surgery: One-Year Follow-Up
Reprinted from: *J. Clin. Med.* **2023**, *12*, 4406, https://doi.org/10.3390/jcm12134406 . . . . **104**

About the Editor

Manuel Wilbring

Prof. Dr. Manuel Wilbring is a distinguished cardiac surgeon and Managing Consultant at the University Heart Center Dresden. Born in 1980 in Bonn, he moved to Dresden in 1993, where he later pursued his medical studies. He began his residency in cardiac surgery in 2007 at the University Heart Center Dresden, with additional training at the University Heart Center Hamburg (2009–2010). He completed his specialization in 2014 and later served as a Senior Consultant at the University Heart Center Halle before returning to Dresden as Managing Consultant.

Prof. Wilbring's clinical and scientific work focuses on minimally invasive cardiac surgery, aortic valve replacement, mitral valve repair, and transcatheter procedures. He has published over 90 peer-reviewed articles on the outcomes of minimally invasive surgery, catheter-based techniques, and the management of infective endocarditis and complex cardiac procedures. As a sought-after speaker, he has delivered over 100 national and international lectures, sharing insights from his research and advancing innovations in modern cardiac surgery.

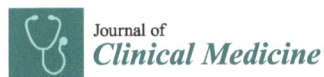
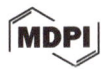

Editorial

Advancing Minimally Invasive Cardiac Surgery—Let's Take a Look into the Future

Manuel Wilbring

Center for Minimally Invasive Cardiac Surgery, University Heart Center Dresden, 01328 Dresden, Germany; manuel.wilbring@gmail.com; Tel.: +49-351-450-1606

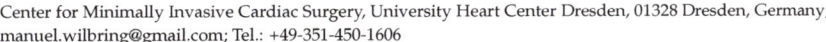

Received: 6 January 2025
Accepted: 16 January 2025
Published: 29 January 2025

Citation: Wilbring, M. Advancing Minimally Invasive Cardiac Surgery—Let's Take a Look into the Future. *J. Clin. Med.* **2025**, *14*, 904. https://doi.org/10.3390/jcm14030904

Copyright: © 2025 by the author. Licensee MDPI, Basel, Switzerland. This article is an open access article distributed under the terms and conditions of the Creative Commons Attribution (CC BY) license (https://creativecommons.org/licenses/by/4.0/).

The evolution of cardiac surgery over the last two decades has been nothing short of revolutionary. Minimally invasive cardiac surgery (MICS) has emerged as a transformative approach, offering patients reduced surgical trauma, faster recovery times, and improved outcomes. Since the pioneering work in minimally invasive cardiac surgery of Rao and Kumar, as well as Sabik and Cosgrove, a continuous process of advancement was set in motion [1–9]. Moreover, the emergence of catheter-based procedures further accelerated the evolution of minimally invasive surgical techniques [10–12].

As cardiac surgeons, we stand at the precipice of a significant paradigm shift. The conventional wisdom that full sternotomy is the gold standard for valve surgery is being increasingly challenged by compelling data supporting MICS. For example, the extensive results from the Dresden group's landmark study on 1000 consecutive patients undergoing transaxillary minimally invasive aortic valve replacement underscore this point [12]. The findings reveal not only the safety and efficacy of this approach but also its potential to become the dominant access route for a wide array of cardiac procedures.

A striking aspect of this transaxillary MICS series is the dramatic increase in its utilization over the study period, rising from 18.7% in 2019 to 97.8% in 2023. This shift signals growing confidence in the technique and reflects the broader trend towards less invasive interventions. Notably, the study demonstrated a 0.9% 30-day mortality rate and a 1.9% rate of major adverse cardiac and cerebrovascular events (MACCEs), reinforcing the notion that transaxillary MICS is not only viable but potentially superior to traditional sternotomy approaches [12].

Several important contributions in this Special Issue further exemplify the advancements and growing scope of MICS: Franz et al. explore the feasibility of minimally invasive mitral valve surgery for patients with infective endocarditis, challenging the notion that this population is unsuitable for less invasive approaches. Salman et al. present hypothermic ventricular fibrillation as a promising strategy for redo mitral valve surgery, addressing the complexities of repeat interventions. Piekarski et al. offer insight into anesthetic protocols critical for ensuring the safety and efficacy of MICS.

Moreover, Taghizadeh-Waghefi et al. focus on the transaxillary approach for high-risk obese patients, demonstrating that MICS can enhance survival and reduce postoperative complications compared to full sternotomy. Ali-Hasan-Al-Saegh et al. likewise delve into the impact of obesity on minimally invasive mitral valve surgery, reinforcing the view that BMI should not limit access to cutting-edge procedures.

Additional articles further enrich the discussion. Moscoso-Ludueña et al. introduce the hybrid concept of combining percutaneous coronary intervention with minimally invasive mitral valve surgery, illustrating the feasibility and safety of this multidisciplinary approach. Meanwhile, Helms et al. emphasize the application of minimally invasive techniques in aortic and hemiarch replacement, underscoring the adaptability of MICS even in complex anatomical scenarios. Kaufeld et al. explore the implications of minimally invasive approaches in thoracic aortic procedures, broadening the scope of this evolving field. Albes et al. provide a comprehensive review on patient selection criteria, offering critical insights into refining procedural indications. Lastly, Weymann et al. present novel data on outcomes following minimally invasive tricuspid valve surgery, further validating the efficacy of MICS across diverse valve pathologies.

Crucially, the success of MICS hinges not only on surgical technique but also on the collaborative efforts of anesthesiologists, perfusionists, and intensive care teams. The Bonn Heart Center protocol for anesthetic management in MICS exemplifies the importance of interdisciplinary coordination in optimizing patient outcomes. Tailored anesthesia protocols, advanced monitoring, and enhanced recovery pathways are essential components that enable the seamless execution of minimally invasive procedures.

The patient-centric benefits of MICS are undeniable. Shorter hospital stays, reduced transfusion requirements, and a faster return to daily activities translate into improved quality of life. A growing body of evidence, including the work by Helms et al. on minimally invasive aortic and hemiarch replacement, suggests that these benefits extend to complex aortic surgeries. This broadens the scope of MICS, reinforcing its role as a cornerstone of modern cardiac surgery.

However, as we embrace the future of MICS, we must also confront the barriers to widespread adoption. The notion that obesity, previous cardiac surgery, or advanced age preclude minimally invasive approaches must be reconsidered. Studies such as those by Ali-Hasan-Al-Saegh et al. demonstrate that obesity is not a contraindication for MICS but rather an opportunity to tailor surgical strategies to individual patient needs. By shifting the focus from patient selection to procedural adaptability, we can expand the reach of MICS and ensure equitable access to its benefits.

In this context, the call to action is clear: "Full sternotomy should soon become an historical access route for valve surgery". This bold assertion reflects the collective sentiment of this Special Issue's contributors, who envision a future where minimally invasive techniques are not reserved for select cases but become the standard of care. The emphasis must shift towards selecting the procedure for the patient, not the patient for the procedure.

The future of minimally invasive valve therapies will increasingly depend on specialized centers, as innovation and excellence in these procedures are best cultivated within dedicated institutions.

In this Special Issue, ten accepted papers highlight the forefront of these advancements in minimally invasive cardiac surgery. The contributions are listed below:

- Taghizadeh-Waghefi, A.; Petrov, A.; Arzt, S.; Alexiou, K.; Matschke, K.; Kappert, U.; Wilbring, M. Minimally Invasive Aortic Valve Replacement for High-Risk Populations: Transaxillary Access Enhances Survival in Patients with Obesity. *J. Clin. Med.* **2024**, *13*, 6529.
- Ali-Hasan-Al-Saegh, S.; Helms, F.; Aburahma, K.; Takemoto, S.; De Manna, N.D.; Amanov, L.; Ius, F.; Karsten, J.; Zubarevich, A.; Schmack, B.; et al. Can obesity serve as a barrier to minimally invasive mitral valve surgery? overcoming the limitations—a multivariate logistic regression analysis. *J. Clin. Med.* **2024**, *13*, 6355.
- Salman, J.; Franz, M.; Aburahma, K.; de Manna, N.D.; Tavil, S.; Ali-Hasan-Al-Saegh, S.; Ius, F.; Boethig, D.; Zubarevich, A.; Schmack, B.; et al. Hypothermic ventricular fibrillation in redo minimally invasive mitral valve surgery: a promising solution for a surgical challenge. *J. Clin. Med.* **2024**, *13*, 4269.

- Franz, M.; Aburahma, K.; Ius, F.; Ali-Hasan-Al-Saegh, S.; Boethig, D.; Hertel, N.; Zubarevich, A.; Kaufeld, T.; Ruhparwar, A.; Weymann, A.; et al. Minimally invasive surgery through right mini-thoracotomy for mitral valve infective endocarditis: contraindicated or safely possible? *J. Clin. Med.* **2024**, *13*, 4182.
- Weymann, A.; Amanov, L.; Beltsios, E.; Arjomandi Rad, A.; Szczechowicz, M.; Merzah, A.S.; Ali-Hasan-Al-Saegh, S.; Schmack, B.; Ismail, I.; Popov, A.-F.; et al. Minimally Invasive Direct Coronary Artery Bypass Grafting: Sixteen Years of Single-Center Experience. *J. Clin. Med.* **2024**, *13*, 3338. https://doi.org/10.3390/jcm13113338.
- Helms, F.; Deniz, E.; Krüger, H.; Zubarevich, A.; Schmitto, J.D.; Poyanmehr, R.; Hinteregger, M.; Martens, A.; Weymann, A.; Ruhparwar, A; Schmack, B.; Popov, A.F. Minimally invasive aortic and hemiarch replacement. *J. Clin. Med.* **2024**, *13*, 4406.
- Moscoso-Ludueña, M.; Vondran, M.; Irqsusi, M.; Nef, H.; Rastan, A.J.; Ghazy, T. Hybrid approach combining PCI and minimally invasive mitral valve surgery. *J. Clin. Med.* **2024**, *13*, 4406.
- Taghizadeh-Waghefi, A.; Petrov, A.; Jatzke, P.; Wilbring, M.; Kappert, U.; Matschke, K.; Alexiou, K.; Arzt, S. Minimally Invasive Isolated Aortic Valve Replacement in a Potential TAVI Cohort of Patients Aged ≥ 75 Years: A Propensity-Matched Analysis. *J. Clin. Med.* **2023**, *12*, 4963. https://doi.org/10.3390/jcm12154963
- Claessens, J.; Goris, P.; Yilmaz, A.; Van Genechten, S.; Claes, M.; Packlé, L.; Pierson, M.; Vandenbrande, J.; Kaya, A.; Stessel, B. Patient-Centred Outcomes after Totally Endoscopic Cardiac Surgery: One-Year Follow-Up. *J. Clin. Med.* **2023**, *12*, 4406. https://doi.org/10.3390/jcm12134406.
- Piekarski, F.; Rohner, M.; Monsefi, N.; Bakhtiary, F.; Velten, M. Anesthesia for minimal invasive cardiac surgery: the bonn heart center protocol. *J. Clin. Med.* **2024**, *13*, 3939.

Conflicts of Interest: The authors declare no conflict of interest.

References

1. Rao, P.N.; Kumar, A.S. Aortic Valve Replacement through Right Thoracotomy. *Tex. Heart Inst. J.* **1993**, *20*, 307–308. [PubMed]
2. Cosgrove, D.M., 3rd.; Sabik, J.F. Minimally Invasive Approach for Aortic Valve Operations. *Ann. Thorac. Surg.* **1996**, *62*, 596–597. [CrossRef] [PubMed]
3. Svensson, L.G.; D'Agostino, R.S. Minimal-Access Aortic and Valvular Operations, Including the "J/j" Incision. *Ann. Thorac. Surg.* **1998**, *66*, 431–435. [CrossRef] [PubMed]
4. Svensson, L.G.; D'Agostino, R.S. "J" Incision Minimal-Access Valve Operations. *Ann. Thorac. Surg.* **1998**, *66*, 1110–1112. [CrossRef] [PubMed]
5. Chang, Y.S.; Lin, P.J.; Chang, C.H.; Chu, J.J.; Tan, P.P. "I" Ministernotomy for Aortic Valve Replacement. *Ann. Thorac. Surg.* **1999**, *68*, 40–45. [CrossRef] [PubMed]
6. Aris, A. Reversed "C" Ministernotomy for Aortic Valve Replacement. *Ann. Thorac. Surg.* **1999**, *67*, 1806–1807. [CrossRef] [PubMed]
7. Loures, D.R.; Mulinari, L.A.; Tyszka, A.L.; Ribeiro, E.; Carvalho, R.G.; Almeida, R. Partial Median Sternotomy in H. A New Approach for Cardiac Surgery. *Arq. Bras. Cardiol.* **1998**, *70*, 71–73. [CrossRef] [PubMed]
8. Lamelas, J. Minimally Invasive Aortic Valve Replacement: The "Miami Method". *Ann. Cardiothorac. Surg.* **2015**, *4*, 71–77. [PubMed]
9. Van Praet, K.M.; Van Kampen, A.; Kofler, M.; Unbehaun, A.; Hommel, M.; Jacobs, S.; Falk, V.; Kempfert, J. Minimally Invasive Surgical Aortic Valve Replacement through a Right Anterolateral Thoracotomy. *Multimed. Man. Cardiothorac. Surg.* **2020**, *2020*, 32436667. [CrossRef] [PubMed]
10. Beckmann, A.; Meyer, R.; Eberhardt, J.; Gummert, J.; Falk, V. German Heart Surgery Report 2023: The Annual Updated Registry of the German Society for Thoracic and Cardiovascular Surgery. *Thorac Cardiovasc Surg.* **2024**, *72*, 329–345. [CrossRef] [PubMed]

11. Coisne, A.; Lancellotti, P.; Habib, G.; Garbi, M.; Dahl, J.S.; Barbanti, M.; Vannan, M.A.; Vassiliou, V.S.; Dudek, D.; Chioncel, O.; et al. ACC/AHA and ESC/EACTS Guidelines for the Management of Valvular Heart Diseases: JACC Guideline Comparison. *J. Am. Coll. Cardiol.* **2023**, *82*, 721–734, Erratum in *J. Am. Coll. Cardiol.* **2023**, *82*, 1648. [CrossRef] [PubMed]
12. Wilbring, M.; Arzt, S.; Taghizadeh-Waghefi, A.; Petrov, A.; Di Eusanio, M.; Matschke, K.; Alexiou, K.; Kappert, U. The transaxillary concept for minimally invasive isolated aortic valve replacement: Results of 1000 consecutive patients. *Eur. J. Cardiothorac. Surg.* **2024**, *66*, ezae427. [CrossRef] [PubMed]

Disclaimer/Publisher's Note: The statements, opinions and data contained in all publications are solely those of the individual author(s) and contributor(s) and not of MDPI and/or the editor(s). MDPI and/or the editor(s) disclaim responsibility for any injury to people or property resulting from any ideas, methods, instructions or products referred to in the content.

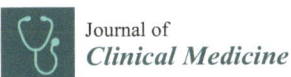

Article

Minimally Invasive Aortic Valve Replacement for High-Risk Populations: Transaxillary Access Enhances Survival in Patients with Obesity

Ali Taghizadeh-Waghefi [1,2,*], Asen Petrov [1,2], Sebastian Arzt [1,2], Konstantin Alexiou [1,2], Klaus Matschke [1,2], Utz Kappert [1,2] and Manuel Wilbring [1,2]

1. Faculty of Medicine Carl Gustav Carus, TU Dresden, 01307 Dresden, Germany
2. Center for Minimally Invasive Cardiac Surgery, University Heart Center Dresden, 01307 Dresden, Germany
* Correspondence: ali.waghefi@gmail.com

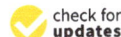

Citation: Taghizadeh-Waghefi, A.; Petrov, A.; Arzt, S.; Alexiou, K.; Matschke, K.; Kappert, U.; Wilbring, M. Minimally Invasive Aortic Valve Replacement for High-Risk Populations: Transaxillary Access Enhances Survival in Patients with Obesity. *J. Clin. Med.* **2024**, *13*, 6529. https://doi.org/10.3390/jcm13216529

Academic Editor: Francesco Pelliccia

Received: 13 September 2024
Revised: 15 October 2024
Accepted: 28 October 2024
Published: 30 October 2024

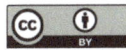

Copyright: © 2024 by the authors. Licensee MDPI, Basel, Switzerland. This article is an open access article distributed under the terms and conditions of the Creative Commons Attribution (CC BY) license (https://creativecommons.org/licenses/by/4.0/).

Abstract: Background/Objectives: Minimally invasive cardiac surgery is often avoided in patients with obesity due to exposure and surgical access concerns. Nonetheless, these patients have elevated periprocedural risks. Minimally invasive transaxillary aortic valve surgery offers a sternum-sparing "nearly no visible scar" alternative to the traditional full sternotomy. This study evaluated the clinical outcomes of patients with obesity compared to a propensity score-matched full sternotomy cohort. **Methods**: This retrospective cohort study included 1086 patients with obesity (body mass index [BMI] of >30 kg/m^2) undergoing isolated aortic valve replacement from 2014 to 2023. Two hundred consecutive patients who received transaxillary minimally invasive cardiac lateral surgery (MICLAT-S) served as a treatment group, while a control group was generated via 1:1 propensity score matching from 886 patients who underwent full sternotomy. The final sample comprised 400 patients in both groups. Outcomes included major adverse cardio-cerebral events, mortality, and postoperative complications. **Results**: After matching, the clinical baselines were comparable. The mean BMI was 34.4 ± 4.0 kg/m^2 (median: 33.9, range: 31.0–64.0). Despite the significantly longer skin-to-skin time (135.0 ± 37.7 vs. 119.0 ± 33.8 min; $p \leq 0.001$), cardiopulmonary bypass time (69.1 ± 19.1 vs. 56.1 ± 21.4 min; $p \leq 0.001$), and aortic cross-clamp time (44.0 ± 13.4 vs. 41.9 ± 13.3 min; $p = 0.044$), the MICLAT-S group showed a shorter hospital stay (9.71 ± 6.19 vs. 12.4 ± 7.13 days; $p \leq 0.001$), lower transfusion requirements (0.54 ± 1.67 vs. 5.17 ± 9.38 units; $p \leq 0.001$), reduced postoperative wound healing issues (5.0% vs. 12.0%; $p = 0.012$), and a lower 30-day mortality rate (1.5% vs. 6.0%; $p = 0.031$). **Conclusions**: MICLAT-S is safe and effective. Compared to traditional sternotomy in patients with obesity, MICLAT-S improves survival, reduces postoperative morbidity, and shortens hospital stays.

Keywords: aortic valve replacement; minimally invasive surgery; transaxillary; MICLAT-S; obesity; BMI; sternum-sparing

1. Introduction

Obesity poses a significant challenge for cardiac surgery, particularly in the context of the current trend toward minimizing surgical trauma and physiological deterioration through minimally invasive techniques. Several publications have reported that the complexities associated with minimally invasive procedures can become a limiting factor for their application in cardiac surgery. Consequently, partly depending on the degree of obesity, patients are often excluded or deselected from these innovative approaches, as obesity is considered a relative contraindication [1,2].

The global prevalence of obesity has reached epidemic proportions. It continues its upward trajectory across nations with varying economic statuses; consequently, the World Health Organization has noted that adult obesity has more than doubled since 1990, while adolescent obesity has even quadrupled [3]. Currently, the prevalence of obesity worldwide is at its highest recorded level and continues to rise [4]. This global obesity epidemic represents a growing challenge for healthcare systems worldwide, which is also reflected in the increasing number of patients with obesity among the cardiac surgical patient population [5]. Furthermore, the demographic shift toward an older population, coupled with an increase in age-related degenerative diseases, has led to a higher prevalence of obesity among patients diagnosed with severe aortic stenosis (AS) [6,7]. Consequently, these patients are increasingly undergoing either surgical aortic valve replacement (SAVR) or transcatheter aortic valve implantation (TAVI) [7]. However, patients with obesity may face additional risks due to their heightened risk profiles and anatomical peculiarities during conventional surgical procedures performed via sternotomy. These patients are at a higher risk of developing deep sternal wound infections following cardiac surgery, along with other complications, such as wound dehiscence, the requirement for prolonged ventilation, and longer hospital stays [8–10]. Nonetheless, mortality following SAVR in patients with obesity remains a contentious topic in the literature, as some studies have reported reduced mortality after cardiac surgery [11]. This unanticipated and seemingly contradictory phenomenon is referred to as the "obesity paradox" [11–13]. This paradox may be explained primarily by selection bias. In risk stratification for elective cardiac surgery, individuals with a high body mass index (BMI) but without metabolic syndrome are more likely to be considered for surgery than those with a higher risk of obesity-related complications [14,15]. Notably, the obesity paradox appears to disappear when evaluating long-term postoperative results, such as the late development of cardiometabolic diseases and the early onset of sternal dehiscence and mediastinitis after sternotomy [16–19]. However, the paradox stands in contrast to findings that identify obesity as an independent predictor of higher hospital mortality [20].

Amid the abovementioned controversies and uncertainties, minimally invasive cardiac surgery (MICS) has gained recognition as a viable alternative aimed at reducing complications and risks, even in high-risk groups. However, it remains unclear whether this promise is substantiated, despite recent advances in MICS. Previous studies have highlighted ongoing uncertainties about the benefits for obese patients, as a smaller incision may result in inadequate surgical field exposure and extended procedure times [21,22]. Furthermore, a large proportion of previous studies on MICS have focused primarily on patients with a lower BMI or an average risk profile. This study sought to fill this gap by investigating the outcomes of MICS–aortic valve replacement (AVR) in obese patients, a group that may be at an elevated risk during surgical procedures. Given the rising rates of obesity and the increasing population of older adults with aortic stenosis, it is essential to establish safe and effective treatment options for these vulnerable groups of patients. In this regard, evaluating MICS as a promising option for patients with obesity and AS can provide valuable insights and potentially influence clinical practice. To date, MICS has not shown any clear survival advantages in the broader population of cardiac surgery patients, likely due to the influence of selection bias. This study evaluated the outcomes of MICS in obese patients, compared to a propensity score-matched cohort who underwent sternotomy.

2. Patients and Methods
2.1. Inclusion and Exclusion Criteria

The main aim of this study was to assess adult patients with obesity undergoing SAVR, specifically comparing those treated with the transaxillary minimally invasive cardiac lateral surgery (MICLAT-S) approach to those treated with a traditional full sternotomy. Obesity was classified as having a BMI greater than 30 kg/m^2. Patients were excluded if they had undergone additional concomitant procedures, had a history of active or recent endocarditis, had previous cardiac surgeries, or did not meet the defined BMI criterion of over 30 kg/m^2.

2.2. Study Design and Ethical Statement

The data for this analysis were gathered retrospectively from electronic health records. The primary outcomes of interest were major adverse cardio-cerebral events (MACCEs), including perioperative myocardial infarction, ischemic stroke, and 30-day mortality. Secondary outcomes included postoperative complications and morbidities. The study protocol received approval from the local ethics committee (EK—Nr. 28092012).

2.3. Patient Population

Between 2014 and 2023, a total of 11,662 patients were included in the Heart Center Database for AVR. Out of these, 2990 patients (28.2%) who underwent concomitant procedures were excluded, along with 850 patients (7.5%) who had endocarditis, redo operations, or emergency surgeries. An additional 5002 patients (40.6%) who underwent transcatheter aortic valve implantation (TAVI) were also excluded, followed by 446 patients (4.6%) who received an upper partial sternotomy and 1288 patients with a body mass index (BMI) below 30 kg/m^2. This left a final cohort of 1086 patients meeting the inclusion criteria. These patients were then divided into two groups: 886 patients (5.4%) who underwent isolated AVR via full median sternotomy and 200 patients (4.6%) who had isolated AVR via the transaxillary MICLAT-S approach. Propensity score matching was applied, resulting in 200 patients in each group for further analysis. The patient selection process is illustrated in the flowchart in Figure 1.

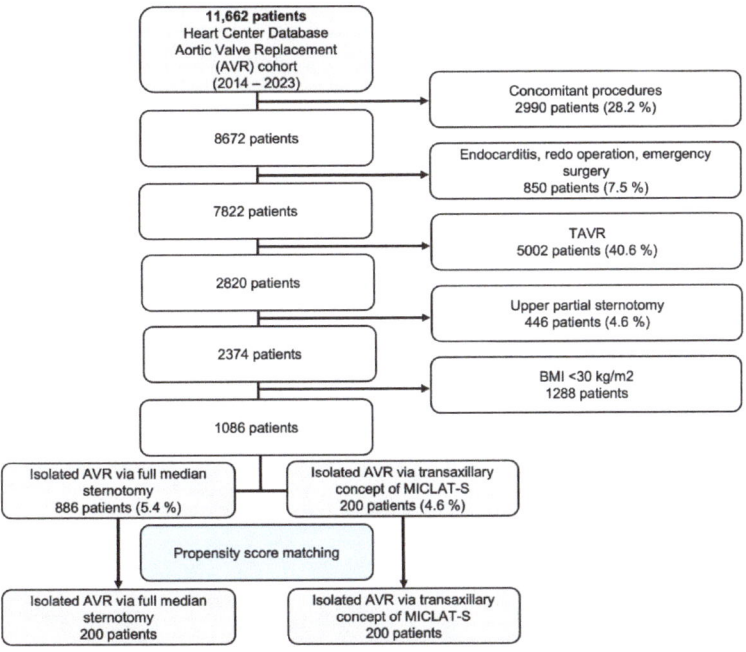

Figure 1. Flow diagram of the study population. TAVR, transcatheter aortic valve replacement; AVR, aortic valve replacement; MICLAT-S, minimally invasive cardiac lateral surgery.

2.4. Involved Surgeons

All MICS-AVR procedures were mainly carried out by four highly experienced surgeons, each with extensive expertise in adult cardiac surgery. Their individual experience with procedures involving extracorporeal circulation ranged from over 500 to 6500 cases. Additionally, based on the structured modular training program and the developments within our surgical team, 64% of the surgical staff were actively involved in performing either the entire procedure or specific parts of it. This involvement stemmed from a well-organized educational approach, where surgical training for residents is divided into linear modules, covering all aspects from femoral vessel preparation to aortic valve surgery. Despite potential confounding factors, such as the transition from selected to all-comer patients and the increased focus on education, these changes have been integrated into the program, resulting in a high level of participation across the surgical team.

2.5. Sternum-Sparing Transaxillary Concept of MICLAT-S

Since the surgical technique for AVR via median sternotomy is well known, it will not be elaborated upon further herein. With the establishment of the MICLAT-S concept at the end of 2019, the year in which the first MICLAT-S approach was implemented, all other MICS approaches—such as upper partial hemisternotomy and right anterolateral thoracotomy—were displaced and outperformed alongside sternotomy. Consequently, by the final year of the study, 97.8% of the AVR procedures were performed using the MICLAT-S approach [23].

For preoperative planning, the anatomical details of the patients were assessed through electrocardiography-gated CT angiography, covering the thoracic, abdominal, and pelvic regions. All patients underwent general anesthesia, and intraoperative transesophageal echocardiography (TEE) was routinely used as the imaging standard, regardless of the surgical technique. In all sternum-sparing MICLAT-S procedures, a double-lumen tube was employed for intubation to allow for single-lung ventilation. Additionally, a temporary transvenous pacing wire was placed via a percutaneous sheath. The femoral vessels were accessed using a conventional surgical cut-down, and extracorporeal circulation was initiated following TEE-guided cannulation. A percutaneous approach for femoral cannulation was only performed if clinical signs of inflammation in the groin area were apparent. Common to all MICS-AVR procedures was the insertion of an antegrade cardioplegia cannula into the ascending aorta, along with the placement of a left ventricular vent line through the right superior pulmonary vein. The method for AVR access via the transaxillary MICLAT-S approach has been described in previous publications. In brief, the patient was positioned supine, with the right side of the chest elevated on two pillows and the right arm resting on the arm support, a position known as the javelin thrower's position (Figure 2). A 5 cm incision was created along the right anterior axillary line, followed by the dissection of the serratus anterior and intercostal muscles to enter the third or fourth intercostal space [24,25]. A video of our AVR procedure using the MICLAT-S technique is available as Supplementary Materials.

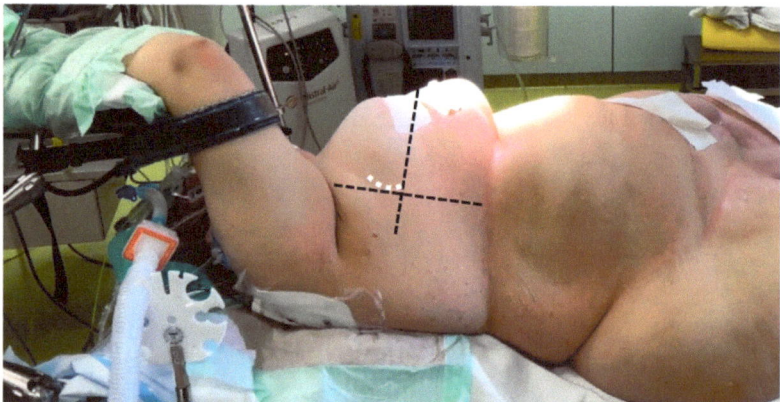

Figure 2. Javelin thrower's position in a female patient with obesity (body mass index = 53.9 kg/m^2). The horizontal dashed line marks the anterior axillary line, while the orthogonal line originates from the mid-sternum (excluding the xiphoid). The white dashed line indicates the incision line.

2.6. Prosthesis Choice

The choice of prosthesis was largely influenced by the surgeon's preference, especially for MICS-AVR procedures. In these cases, comprehensive anatomical information was obtained through a high-resolution, full cardiac cycle CT scan, following the TAVI-CT protocol, covering the thorax, abdomen, and pelvis. This scan provided important preoperative data, including measurements such as the distance from the annular plane to the chest wall, the size of the aortic annulus, and the anticipated valve size. These measurements played a key role in the surgeon's decision-making process. With growing evidence supporting the durability of rapid deployment valves (RDVs), their use was not restricted [26–28].

2.7. Statistical Analysis

The Shapiro–Wilk test was used to check if continuous variables followed a normal distribution. For those that did, a *t*-test was applied, while the Mann–Whitney U test was used for non-normally distributed variables and those on ordinal scales. Fisher's exact test and the chi-square test were employed to analyze dichotomous and other categorical variables, respectively.

Propensity score matching was conducted to address baseline imbalances between the groups, considering factors such as age, sex, EuroSCORE II, BMI, left ventricular ejection fraction (LVEF), atrial fibrillation, peripheral vascular disease, chronic kidney disease, and chronic lung disease. Since corrections for type I errors were not implemented for multiple comparisons, the inferential statistical results serve a descriptive purpose, with significance indicated by a local *p*-value below 0.05, without implying an error rate under 5%. All statistical analyses were performed using the open-source R software (version 4.4.1).

3. Results

3.1. Baseline Patient Characteristics

From January 2014 to February 2023, a total of 1086 patients underwent surgery, with 886 receiving a sternotomy and 200 undergoing MICLAT-S. Several significant differences in the baseline demographic and clinical characteristics were observed between the two groups. The sternotomy group tended to be older ($p = 0.034$), while the MICLAT-S group more frequently had atrial fibrillation ($p = 0.021$). Additionally, the sternotomy group showed a higher prevalence of diabetes mellitus ($p = 0.038$) and peripheral arterial occlusive disease ($p = 0.004$). The MICLAT-S group was significantly more likely to have had a transient ischemic attack ($p < 0.001$). However, there were no significant differences concerning the BMI, LVEF, or EuroSCORE II. A significant difference was noted in the prevalence of pulmonary arterial hypertension, which was considerably more common in the sternotomy group ($p < 0.001$).

Propensity scores, based on the defined variables, were applied to match 200 patients from each group within the full cohort, ensuring comparable baseline characteristics between them. After matching, there was clear alignment in the baseline characteristics across both groups. Table 1 provides an overview of the baseline characteristics for both the unmatched and propensity score-matched groups.

Table 1. Baseline characteristics.

	Pre-Matched Cohort			Propensity Score-Matched Cohort		
	Sternotomy (n = 886)	MICLAT-S (n = 200)	p	Sternotomy (n = 200)	MICLAT-S (n = 200)	p
Age (year), mean ± SD	69.0 ± 8.65	67.6 ± 8.27	*0.034* *	68.4 ± 8.25	67.6 ± 8.27	0.327
BMI (kg/m^2), mean ± SD	33.8 ± 3.43	34.1 ± 3.76	0.205	34.6 ± 4.21	34.1 ± 3.76	0.227
Diabetes mellitus, n (%)	379 (42.8)	69 (35.5)	*0.038* *	75 (37.5)	69 (34.5)	0.603
Previous MI, n (%)	24 (2.7)	6 (3.0)	1	8 (4.0)	6 (3.0)	0.787
LVEF > 50%, n (%)	671 (75.7)	155 (77.5)	0.156	159 (79.5)	155 (77.5)	0.948
Atrial fibrillation, n (%)	107 (12.1)	37 (18.5)	*0.021* *	48 (24.0)	37 (18.5)	0.221
COPD, n (%)	75 (8.5)	24 (12.0)	0.152	31 (15.5)	24 (12.0)	0.384
Renal insufficiency, n (%)	243 (27.4)	48 (24.0)	0.368	53 (26.5)	48 (24.0)	0.645
Hemodialysis, n (%)	7 (0.8)	4 (2.0)	0.249	4 (2.0)	4 (2.0)	1
PAOD, n (%)	126 (14.2)	13 (6.5)	*0.004* **	17 (8.5)	13 (6.5)	0.570
TIA, n (%)	0 (0)	4 (2.0)	*<0.001* **	0 (0)	4 (2.0)	0.123
EuroSCORE II (%), mean ± SD	1.68 ± 1.24	1.83 ± 1.21	0.286	1.83 ± 1.81	1.83 ± 1.21	0.989

Bold and italic values indicate statistical significance: * $p \leq 0.05$; ** $p \leq 0.01$; MICLAT-S, minimally invasive cardiac lateral surgery; SD, standard deviation; BMI, body mass index; LVEF, left ventricular ejection fraction; COPD, chronic obstructive pulmonary disease; PAOD, peripheral arterial occlusive disease; TIA, transient ischemic attack.

3.2. Unadjusted Outcomes

3.2.1. Procedural and Intraoperative Data

Among the pre-matched cohort, the prosthesis size was significantly larger in the MICLAT-S group (24.2 ± 2.1 mm) than in the sternotomy group (23.2 ± 1.8 mm; $p \leq 0.001$; Table 2). Regarding the prosthesis type, RDVs were used in 81.9% of the patients in the MICLAT-S group, while none were used in the sternotomy group. Bioprosthetic and mechanical valves were significantly more commonly used in the sternotomy group (84.7% vs. 13.4%; $p \leq 0.001$; 15.3% vs. 4.7%, respectively; Figure 3; Table 2). The MICLAT-S group also exhibited a significantly longer skin-to-skin time (STST) (135.0 ± 37.7 vs. 120.1 ± 33.6 min; $p \leq 0.001$), cardiopulmonary bypass time (CPBT) (69.1 ± 19.1 vs. 59.2 ± 23.5 min; $p \leq 0.001$), and aortic cross-clamp time (ACCT) (44.0 ± 13.4 vs. 41.9 ± 15.2 min; $p = 0.044$; Figure 4; Table 2).

Table 2. Procedural and intraoperative data.

	Pre-Matched Cohort			Propensity Score-Matched Cohort		
	Sternotomy (n = 886)	MICLAT-S (n = 200)	p	Sternotomy (n = 200)	MICLAT-S (n = 200)	p
Prosthesis size (mm), mean ± SD	23.2 ± 1.8	24.2 ± 2.1	*≤0.001* **	23.7 ± 1.9	24.1 ± 2.0	*0.041* *
STST (min), mean ± SD	120.1 ± 33.6	135.0 ± 37.7	*≤0.001* **	119.0 ± 33.8	135.0 ± 37.7	*≤0.001* **
CPBT (min), mean ± SD	59.2 ± 23.5	69.1 ± 19.1	*≤0.001* **	56.1 ± 21.4	69.1 ± 19.1	*≤0.001* **
ACCT (min), mean ± SD	41.9 ± 15.2	44.0 ± 13.4	*0.044* *	41.9 ± 13.3	44.0 ± 13.4	*0.044* *
Prosthesis type						
- Mechanical, n (%)	136 (15.3)	10 (5.0)		29 (14.5)	10 (5.0)	
- Bioprosthetic, n (%)	750 (84.7)	21 (10.5)	*≤0.001* **	171 (85.5)	21 (10.5)	*≤0.001* **
- RDV, n (%)	0 (0.0)	169 (84.5)		0 (0.0)	169 (84.5)	

Bold and italic values indicate statistical significance: * $p \leq 0.05$; ** $p \leq 0.01$; MICLAT-S, minimally invasive cardiac lateral surgery; SD, standard deviation; min, minute; STST, skin-to-skin time; CPBT, cardiopulmonary bypass time; ACCT, aortic cross-clamp time; RDV, rapid deployment valve.

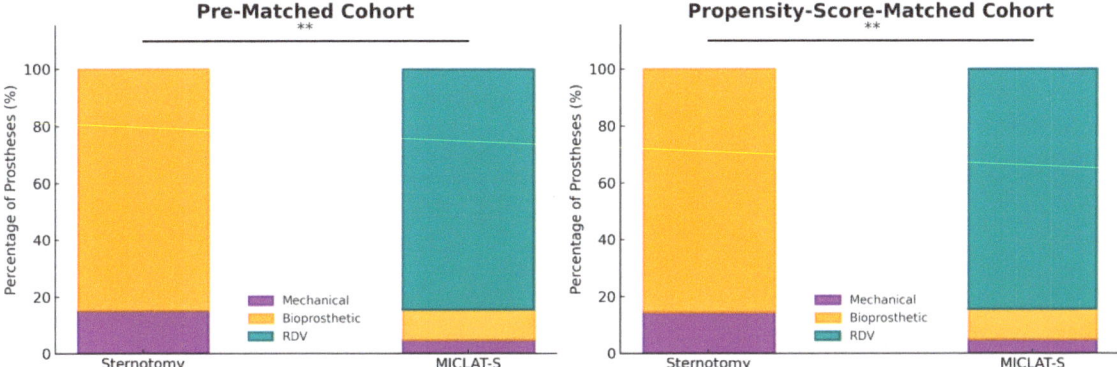

Figure 3. Distribution of the type of aortic valve prostheses implanted within each group. MICLAT-S, minimally invasive cardiac lateral surgery; RDV, rapid deployment valve; ** $p \leq 0.01$.

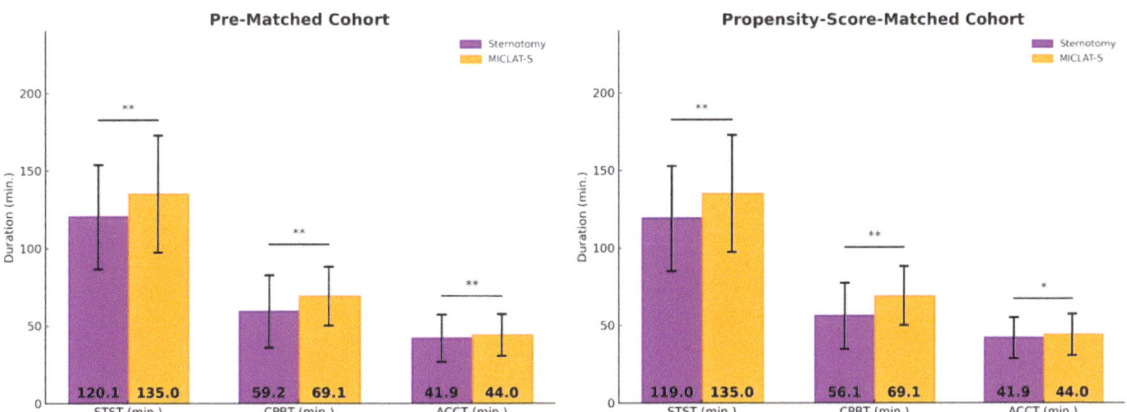

Figure 4. Surgical times. * $p < 0.05$ between groups; MICLAT-S, minimally invasive cardiac lateral surgery; min, minute; STST, skin-to-skin time; CPBT, cardiopulmonary bypass time; ACCT, aortic cross-clamp time; * $p \leq 0.05$; ** $p \leq 0.01$.

3.2.2. Postoperative Outcomes, Morbidity, and Mortality

Among the pre-matched cohort, significant differences were observed in several key postoperative outcomes between the MICLAT-S and sternotomy groups. A ventilation time of ≤12 h was significantly more common in the MICLAT-S group than in the sternotomy group (90.5% vs. 26.2%; $p \leq 0.001$). Regarding the intensive care unit (ICU) stay, the MICLAT-S group demonstrated a shorter duration, with 70.5% of the patients staying ≤24 h, compared to 57.7% in the sternotomy group ($p = 0.006$). Likewise, the overall hospital stay was notably shorter in the MICLAT-S group (9.71 ± 6.19 vs. 12.6 ± 8.60 days; $p \leq 0.001$). The MICLAT-S group required significantly fewer packed red blood cell transfusions, with an average of 0.54 ± 1.67 units, compared to 4.02 ± 7.37 units in the sternotomy group ($p \leq 0.001$). Although the incidence of acute kidney injury (AKI) stage III or continuous veno-venous hemofiltration (CVVH) was lower in the MICLAT-S group (2.0% vs. 5.0%), this difference did not reach statistical significance ($p = 0.097$). However, the re-exploration rates were significantly higher in the MICLAT-S group (6.5% vs. 3.2%; $p = 0.043$). There was no significant difference between the groups in the incidence of wound healing complications and postoperative delirium. The incidence of both ischemic and disabling strokes was comparable between the groups. Additionally, the 30-day mortality rate was lower in the MICLAT-S group, although the difference was not statistically significant (1.5% vs. 3.4%; p = 0.240). Lastly, MACCEs were significantly less common in the MICLAT-S group than in the sternotomy group (2.0% vs. 5.1%; p = 0.028). The results for the postoperative parameters for the pre-matched cohort can be found in Table 3.

Table 3. Postoperative morbidity and mortality.

	Pre-Matched Cohort			Propensity Score-Matched Cohort		
	Sternotomy (n = 886)	MICLAT-S (n = 200)	p	Sternotomy (n = 200)	MICLAT-S (n = 200)	p
Ventilation time (h)						
- ≤12, n (%)	232 (26.2)	181 (90.5)	≤*0.001* **	47 (23.5)	181 (90.5)	≤*0.001* **
- ≤24, n (%)	525 (59.3)	13 (6.5)		139 (69.5)	13 (6.5)	
- >24, n (%)	57 (6.4)	6 (3.0)		14 (7.0)	6 (3.0)	
Respiratory failure [†], n (%)	40 (4.5)	6 (3.0)	0.442	11 (5.5)	6 (3.0)	0.322
ICU stay (days), mean ± SD						
- ≤24, n (%)	511 (57.7)	141 (70.5)		120 (60.0)	141 (70.5)	
- ≤48, n (%)	133 (15.0)	17 (8.5)	*0.006* **	27 (13.5)	17 (8.5)	0.068
- <72, n (%)	89 (10.0)	21 (10.5)		19 (9.5)	21 (10.5)	
- >72, n (%)	152 (17.2)	21 (10.5)		34 (17.0)	21 (10.5)	
Hospital stay (days), mean ± SD	12.6 ± 8.60	9.71 ± 6.19	≤*0.001* **	12.4 ± 7.13	9.71 ± 6.19	≤*0.001* **
Transfusion of PRBCs, mean ± SD	4.02 ± 7.37	0.540 ± 1.67	≤*0.001* **	5.17 ± 9.38	0.540 ± 1.67	≤*0.001* **
AKI stage III or CVVH, n (%)	44 (5.0)	4 (2.0)	0.097	18 (9.0)	4 (2.0)	*0.022* *
Conversion to sternotomy, n (%)	N/A	7 (1.6)	N/A	N/A	7 (1.6)	N/A
Re-exploration, n (%)	28 (3.2)	13 (6.5)	*0.043* *	5 (2.5)	13 (6.5)	0.0888
Impaired wound healing, n (%)	53 (6.0)	10 (5.0)	0.707	24 (12.0)	10 (5.0)	*0.012* **
Postoperative delirium, n (%)	157 (17.7)	40 (20.0)	0.517	26 (13.0)	40 (20.0)	0.0794
Ischemic stroke (Rankin ≥ 2), n (%)	12 (1.4)	1 (0.5)	0.490	2 (1.0)	1 (0.5)	0.745
TIA, n (%)	9 (1.0)	1 (0.5)	0.745	2 (1.0)	1 (0.5)	0.618
PPM implantation, n (%)	4 (0.5)	11 (5.5)	0.446	1 (0.5)	11 (5.5)	1
Myocardial infarction, n (%)	4 (0.5)	0 (0.0)	0.758	1 (0.5)	0 (0)	1
30-day mortality, n (%)	30 (3.4)	3 (1.5)	0.240	12 (6.0)	3 (1.5)	*0.031* *
MACCE, n (%)	45 (5.1)	4 (2.0)	*0.028* *	15 (7.5)	4 (2.0)	*0.003* **

Bold and italic values indicate statistical significance: * $p \leq 0.05$; ** $p \leq 0.01$; [†] Primary postoperative ventilation time of ≥72 h, reintubation, and tracheotomy; MICLAT-S, minimally invasive cardiac lateral surgery; SD, standard deviation; ICU, intensive care unit; PRBC, packed red blood cell; AKI, acute kidney injury; CVVH, continuous veno-venous hemofiltration; TIA, transient ischemic attack; PPM, permanent pacemaker; N/A, not applicable.

3.3. Propensity Score-Matched Cohort

To mitigate the influence of potential confounding variables, we applied propensity score matching between the two groups, resulting in 400 patients (200 matched pairs) for further analysis.

3.3.1. Adjusted Procedural and Intraoperative Data

Among the propensity score-matched cohort, the prosthesis size remained significantly larger in the MICLAT-S group (24.1 ± 2.0 vs. 23.7 ± 1.9 mm; p = 0.041; Table 2). The prosthesis type distribution remained consistent with the pre-matched cohort. RDVs were used in 84.5% of the patients in the MICLAT-S group, while none were used in the sternotomy group. Bioprosthetic and mechanical valves were significantly more commonly used in the sternotomy group (85.5% vs. 10.5%; $p \leq 0.001$; 14.5% vs. 5.0%, respectively; Figure 3; Table 2). The MICLAT-S group continued to show a significantly longer STST (135.0 ± 37.7 vs. 119.0 ± 33.8 min; $p \leq 0.001$), CPBT (69.1 ± 19.1 vs. 56.1 ± 21.4 min; $p \leq 0.001$), and ACCT (44.0 ± 13.4 vs. 41.9 ± 13.3 min; p = 0.044; Figure 4; Table 2).

3.3.2. Adjusted Postoperative Outcomes, Morbidity, and Mortality

Within the matched cohort, the MICLAT-S group continued to demonstrate significant advantages. The proportion of patients requiring ventilation for ≤12 h remained significantly larger in the MICLAT-S group (90.5%) than in the sternotomy group (23.5%) ($p \leq 0.001$; Figure 5). The trend of shorter ICU stays seen in the unmatched cohort did not achieve statistical significance in the matched cohort, although it did show a statistical tendency (70.5% of the patients in the MICLAT-S group vs. 60.0% of those in the sternotomy group stayed ≤24 h; $p = 0.068$; Figure 5). However, the overall hospital stay, which was significantly shorter in the MICLAT-S group in the unmatched cohort, remained significantly reduced among the matched cohort (9.71 ± 6.19 vs. 12.4 ± 7.13 days; $p \leq 0.001$; Figure 6). In alignment with the unmatched cohort findings, the MICLAT-S group among the matched cohort required significantly fewer transfusions of packed red blood cells (0.54 ± 1.67 vs. 5.17 ± 9.38 units; $p \leq 0.001$). The lower incidence of AKI stage III or postoperative-onset CVVH was confirmed in the matched cohort (2.0% vs. 9.0%; $p = 0.022$). The re-exploration rates, which were significantly higher in the MICLAT-S group among the unmatched cohort, remained elevated among the matched cohort (6.5% vs. 2.5%) but did not reach statistical significance ($p = 0.089$). Conversely, the trend of reduced wound healing complications in the MICLAT-S group continued and became statistically significant in the matched cohort (5.0% vs. 12.0%; $p = 0.012$). Although postoperative delirium syndrome occurred more frequently in the MICLAT-S group in both the unmatched and matched cohorts, the difference was not statistically significant in the matched cohort (20.0% vs. 13.0%; $p = 0.0794$). Notably, the difference in the 30-day mortality rate, which was not statistically significant among the unmatched cohort, became significant after propensity score matching, with the MICLAT-S group showing a lower rate (1.5% vs. 6.0%; $p = 0.031$). Moreover, the propensity score matching reinforced the significantly lower incidence of MACCEs in the MICLAT-S group (2.0% vs. 7.5%; $p = 0.003$). Postoperative outcomes for the propensity score-matched cohort are detailed in Table 3.

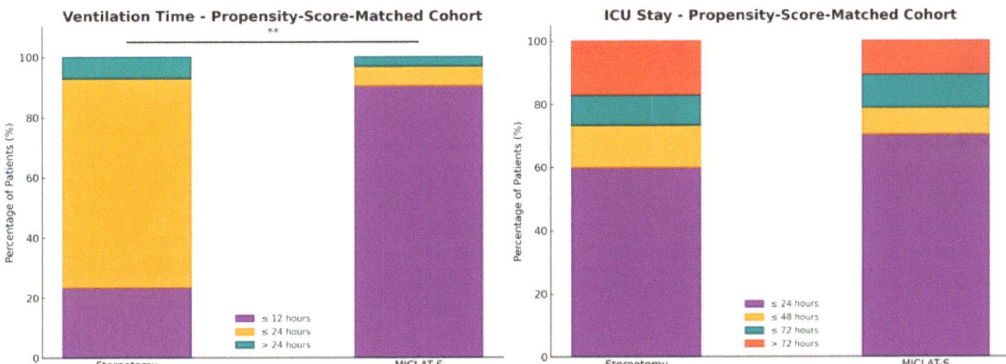

Figure 5. Two stacked bar charts present the percentage distribution of patients in the propensity score-matched cohort for both the ventilation time (on the left) and ICU stay (on the right). Each bar represents the percentage of patients in each group who experienced different durations of ventilation (min) or ICU stays (day). The stacked bars for both the sternotomy and MICLAT-S groups total 100%, representing the total distribution of patients across the different time intervals; ** $p \leq 0.01$.

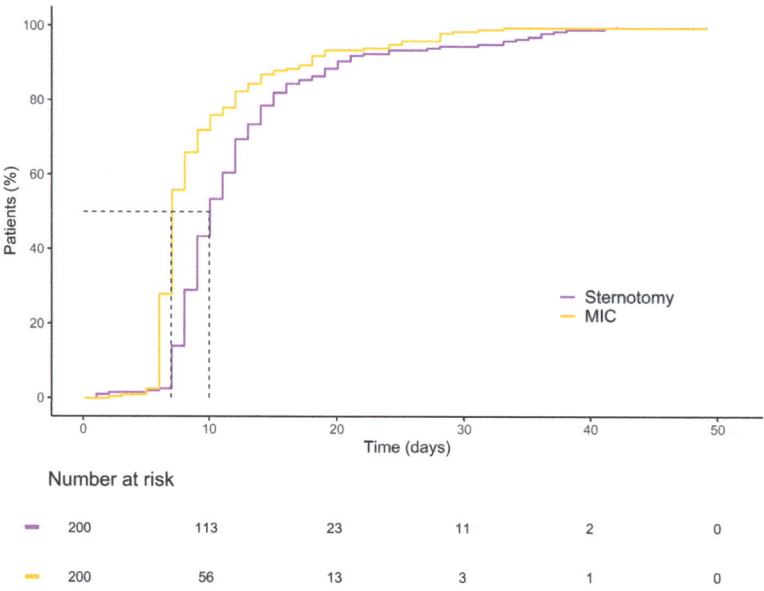

Figure 6. Kaplan–Meier curve illustrating the cumulative probability of patients remaining hospitalized over time for each group.

4. Discussion

Minimally invasive techniques for AVR have evolved significantly over the past three decades, with sternum-sparing approaches emerging even before the introduction of the upper partial hemisternotomy. In the 1990s, pioneering efforts by Rao and Kumar (1993) and Cosgrove and Sabik (1996) laid the groundwork for sternum-sparing approaches in MICS-AVR [29,30]. Notably, Cosgrove advanced the field by reducing thoracic trauma through the incorporation of femoral cannulation in MICS-AVR [30]. The introduction of MICS-AVR via upper partial hemisternotomy by Svensson in 1997 marked another milestone [31]. However, before the widespread clinical adoption of TAVI, MICS-AVR accounted for less than 5% of all cases in Germany [28]. The growing awareness of and emphasis on reducing surgical invasiveness, spurred by the advent of TAVI, ultimately led to a renaissance for sternum-sparing techniques, exemplified by the development of RAT by Lamelas in 2015 [32]. This approach was further refined with the introduction of the endoscopically guided right anterolateral thoracotomy in 2020 [33].

After nearly 30 years of development, the current state of cardiac surgery in the treatment of aortic valve pathologies presents a rather sobering conclusion. Despite innovations, the adoption of sternum-sparing techniques remains notably low, and they are not even mentioned in the annual German Heart Surgery Reports [29]. Additionally, while the upper partial hemisternotomy for AVR remains the most commonly used minimally invasive technique, its adoption has increased but still remains below 50%; it is currently at 43.2% [34]. This suggests that most patients undergoing treatment for aortic valve pathologies still undergo a conventional full sternotomy. Notably, the adoption rate of minimally invasive procedures for isolated AVR is low, and there is ongoing hesitancy regarding their use. A plausible explanation is that the minimally invasive techniques developed thus far carry an inherent limitation, restricting their applicability to a highly selective patient cohort [35]. This high degree of selectivity hinders the establishment of an evidence-based foundation for the application of minimally invasive techniques across the broader all-comer patient population. It also creates clinical bias by selecting lower-risk patients for minimally invasive procedures, which in turn leads to insufficient statistical power to show a significant reduction in mortality compared to the median sternotomy approach; this is particularly relevant as no studies to date have demonstrated a clear mortality benefit for MICS in the broader cardiac surgery population [21,36–39].

To the best of our knowledge, our study is the first to present evidence from a substantial cohort of 1086 patients, showing that individuals with obesity and undergoing MICS-AVR experience significantly better survival and reduced postoperative morbidity than a propensity score-matched sternotomy cohort. The main results of this study are as follows:

- Combined MACCEs were less frequently observed in the MICLAT-S group;
- The postoperative 30-day mortality rate was significantly lower in the MICLAT-S group;
- The MICLAT-S group had a shorter median hospital stay;
- The incidence of postoperative impaired wound healing was significantly lower in the MICLAT-S group;
- The MICLAT-S group needed fewer transfusions of blood products.

Patients with obesity have been excluded from major reports on minimally invasive valve surgery, which is why comparative studies are scarce. The right anterolateral thoracotomy, as a sternum-sparing approach for AVR, has so far only been examined in small case series comparing valve surgeries to sternotomy or in comparative studies with limited patient numbers [40,41]. Further studies have investigated the upper partial hemisternotomy as a minimally invasive option, comparing it to a median sternotomy in obese patients [42–48]. However, these studies have not provided evidence of the superiority of MICS techniques over conventional methods in terms of mortality for isolated AVR. Among the defined primary endpoints in the present study, while the incidence of perioperative stroke and myocardial infarction was comparable between the two groups, that of both 30-day mortality and MACCEs was significantly lower in the MICLAT-S group than in the sternotomy group. These findings confirm that the transaxillary concept of MICLAT-S, as a sternum-sparing MICS-AVR technique, outperforms the conventional full median sternotomy for AVR in patients with obesity. Notably, throughout the study period, the selection of patients for the MICLAT-S approach was entirely independent of anthropometric factors.

In terms of hospital resource utilization, the MICLAT-S group demonstrated clear superiority. The MICLAT-S group experienced notably shorter ventilation times and overall hospital stays compared to the control group. After matching, only a statistical trend was observed regarding shorter ICU stays in the MICLAT-S group. This observation is consistent with the findings of other studies that compared MICS procedures to sternotomy in patients with obesity for isolated AVR [40,43–46,49,50]. A possible explanation for the shorter hospital stays could be that the MICLAT-S technique, which is bone-sparing and avoids affecting the shoulder girdle, may enable earlier patient mobilization and accelerated recovery, leading to quicker patient independence and earlier discharge. However, this hypothesis requires further validation in future studies. Moreover, consistent with previous reports, the MICLAT-S group required significantly fewer perioperative transfusions of packed red blood cells [40,42,45,46,51].

One drawback of the minimally invasive procedure was the extended procedural duration, which included a longer surgical time, CPBT, and cross-clamp time. However, this did not have any clinically apparent impact on the primary endpoints or other postoperative morbidities. On the contrary, the need for perioperative transfusions and the incidence of acute renal failure and postoperative new-onset dialysis were lower in the MICS-AVR group. While the lower incidence of acute renal failure in the MICLAT-S group, despite longer procedural times, might seem surprising, the most plausible explanation lies in the significantly fewer complications and reduced transfusion requirements in the minimally invasive group—both of which are key contributors to the development of renal failure [40,52].

RDVs were exclusively implanted in the MICLAT-S group, consistent with previous reports and likely explaining the implantation of larger valve prostheses in this cohort [53].

In the MICLAT-S group, seven patients (1.6%) underwent conversion to sternotomy. However, none of these conversions were attributed to inadequate exposure of the aortic valve.

As anticipated, the occurrence of thoracic wound healing complications was significantly higher in the sternotomy group than in the MICLAT-S group. The groups differed not only in the incidence but also in the location of such disorders. In the MICLAT-S group, wound healing complications predominantly arose at the groin (60%, $n/N = 6/10$) and were less common in the thoracic area (40%, $n/N = 4/10$), whereas, in the control group, they were exclusively localized to the sternum. Notably, 45.8% ($n/N = 11/24$) of the patients with sternal wound healing disorders in the control group developed consequent mediastinitis. In contrast, no cases of mediastinitis were observed in the MICLAT-S group. Among the cases of local wound healing disorders in the groin, 66.7% ($n/N = 4/6$) were primarily attributed to the formation of a lymph fistula, while the remaining cases had a primary infection of the groin wound.

Finally, the cosmetic outcomes of the transaxillary concept of MICLAT-S were particularly satisfactory, especially in the female patients with obesity, due to the minimized visibility of scars and the sternum-sparing nature of the procedure (Figure 7).

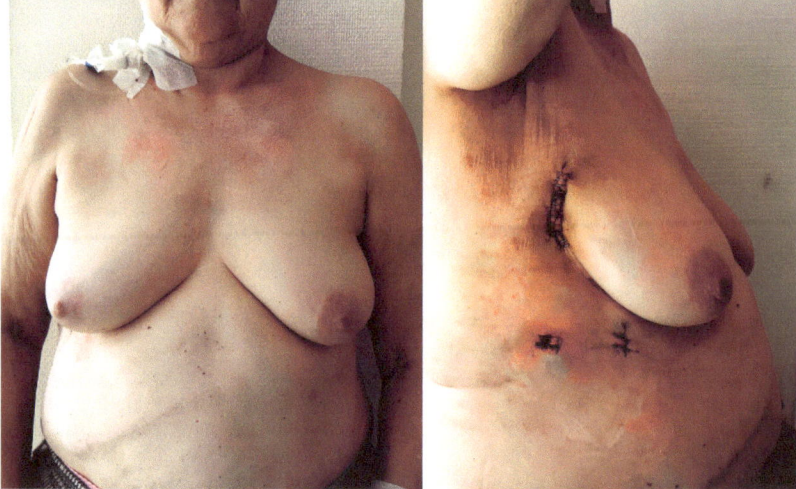

Figure 7. Postoperative cosmetic outcomes of minimally invasive cardiac lateral surgery in a female patient with obesity (body mass index of 31.1 kg/m^2). The images illustrate the minimally invasive nature of the procedure. The sternum remains intact, and the incisions are placed in the right anterior axillary line, minimizing visible scarring, particularly in female patients with a higher body mass index. The right image demonstrates the primary surgical incision, contributing to enhanced cosmetic outcomes and more comfortable postoperative recovery.

5. Conclusions

The results underscore the potential of the holistic transaxillary concept of MICLAT-S as a viable, more broadly applicable alternative to traditional sternotomy, particularly in patients with obesity. Given the limited research on minimally invasive techniques, especially sternum-sparing procedures, this study provides crucial evidence that could pave the way for the broader adoption and further exploration of these approaches in this challenging patient population. Furthermore, the results of this study offer a strong basis for the hypothesis that minimally invasive procedures, when extended beyond the confines of highly selective patient cohorts and applied as a therapeutic strategy for the broader all-comer population, have the potential to confer significant advantages, even in high-risk and high-morbidity patient groups. Consequently, the overarching goal of minimally invasive techniques should not be limited by the specific method of implementation but should instead focus on making them accessible to the entire spectrum of cardiac surgical patients. Therefore, it is not the patient who must be deemed suitable for the MICS approach, but rather the MICS approach that must be adapted to meet the needs of all patients. While TAVI is seeking to further expand its evidence base from high- to intermediate- and low-risk patients, MICS-AVR remains predominantly in the domain of low-risk patients. One reason that an all-comer approach has so far failed to gain widespread acceptance for MICS-AVR in cardiac surgery centers is the lack of a holistic concept. Therefore, the emerging generation of cardiac surgeons must address the areas of greatest need, breaking the paradigm of offering minimally invasive procedures only to low-risk patients and extending MICS to all risk groups, regardless of their morbidity profile. Immediate efforts should be directed toward integrating these findings into clinical practice, ensuring that the benefits of MICLAT-S are made available to a broader range of patients, thereby advancing the field of cardiac surgery as a whole.

6. Limitations

This study has several limitations. First, although the cohort was large, the research was conducted at a single center and was a retrospective analysis with a relatively short follow-up period. Second, the propensity score matching model may have missed unknown but potentially important risk factors and confounding variables. Third, the matching criteria were mainly chosen based on the surgical feasibility of minimally invasive AVR. Finally, the outcomes were obtained in a high-volume, specialized center, which may reduce the generalizability of the findings to wider patient populations.

Supplementary Materials: The following supporting information can be downloaded at: https://zenodo.org/records/13760664; Minimally Invasive Transaxillary Approach: Aortic Valve Replacement in a Patient with BMI > 50 kg/m^2.

Author Contributions: Conceptualization, M.W. and U.K.; methodology, M.W. and A.P.; software, M.W., A.P. and A.T.-W.; validation, U.K., K.A. and K.M.; formal analysis, A.P.; investigation, A.P. and A.T.-W.; resources, K.A. and S.A.; data curation, S.A., A.P. and A.T.-W.; writing—original draft preparation, A.T.-W.; writing—review and editing, U.K. and M.W.; visualization, A.P. and A.T.-W.; supervision, K.M.; project administration, U.K. and K.M. All authors have read and agreed to the published version of the manuscript.

Funding: This research received no external funding.

Institutional Review Board Statement: This study was conducted in accordance with the Declaration of Helsinki and approved by the Ethics Committee at the Technical University of Dresden (protocol code EK-28092012, granted in September 2012).

Informed Consent Statement: Patient consent was waived due to the retrospective nature of the study, with anonymized data and no direct patient interaction.

Data Availability Statement: The data presented in this study are available on request from the corresponding author. The data are not publicly available due to ethical regulations.

Conflicts of Interest: The authors declare no conflicts of interest.

References

1. Gammie, J.S.; Bartlett, S.T.; Griffith, B.P. Small-incision mitral valve repair: Safe, durable, and approaching perfection. *Ann. Surg.* **2009**, *250*, 409–415. [CrossRef] [PubMed]
2. Müller, L.; Höfer, D.; Holfeld, J.; Hangler, H.; Bonaros, N.; Grimm, M. Indications and contra-indications for minimally invasive mitral valve surgery. *J. Vis. Surg.* **2018**, *4*, 255. [CrossRef]
3. WHO (World Health Organization). Obesity and Overweight. 2024. Available online: https://www.who.int/news-room/fact-sheets/detail/obesity-and-overweight (accessed on 25 May 2024).
4. NCD Risk Factor Collaboration (NCD-RisC). Worldwide trends in body-mass index, underweight, overweight, and obesity from 1975 to 2016: A pooled analysis of 2416 population-based measurement studies in 128.9 million children, adolescents, and adults. *Lancet* **2017**, *390*, 2627–2642. [CrossRef] [PubMed]

5. Brinkman, W.T.; Hoffman, W.; Dewey, T.M.; Culica, D.; Prince, S.L.; Herbert, M.A.; Mack, M.J.; Ryan, W.H. Aortic valve replacement surgery: Comparison of outcomes in matched sternotomy and PORT ACCESS groups. *Ann. Thorac. Surg.* 2010, *90*, 131–135. [CrossRef]
6. McInerney, A.; Rodes-Cabau, J.; Veiga, G.; Lopez-Otero, D.; Munoz-Garcia, E.; Campelo-Parada, F.; Oteo, J.F.; Carnero, M.; Tafur Soto, J.D.; Amat-Santos, I.J.; et al. Transcatheter versus surgical aortic valve replacement in patients with morbid obesity: A multicentre propensity score-matched analysis. *EuroIntervention* 2022, *18*, e417–e427. [CrossRef]
7. McInerney, A.; Tirado-Conte, G.; Rodes-Cabau, J.; Campelo-Parada, F.; Tafur Soto, J.D.; Barbanti, M.; Munoz-Garcia, E.; Arif, M.; Lopez, D.; Toggweiler, S.; et al. Impact of morbid obesity and obesity phenotype on outcomes after transcatheter aortic valve replacement. *J. Am. Heart Assoc.* 2021, *10*, e019051. [CrossRef]
8. Yap, C.H.; Mohajeri, M.; Yii, M. Obesity and early complications after cardiac surgery. *Med. J. Aust.* 2007, *186*, 350–354. [CrossRef]
9. Ghanta, R.K.; LaPar, D.J.; Zhang, Q.; Devarkonda, V.; Isbell, J.M.; Yarboro, L.T.; Kern, J.A.; Kron, I.L.; Speir, A.M.; Fonner, C.E.; et al. Obesity increases risk-adjusted morbidity, mortality, and cost following cardiac surgery. *J. Am. Heart Assoc.* 2017, *6*, e003831. [CrossRef]
10. Allama, A.; Ibrahim, I.; Abdallah, A.; Ashraf, S.; Youhana, A.; Kumar, P.; Bhatti, F.; Zaidi, A. Effect of body mass index on early clinical outcomes after cardiac surgery. *Asian Cardiovasc. Thorac. Ann.* 2014, *22*, 667–673. [CrossRef]
11. Stamou, S.C.; Nussbaum, M.; Stiegel, R.M.; Reames, M.K.; Skipper, E.R.; Robicsek, F.; Lobdell, K.W. Effect of body mass index on outcomes after cardiac surgery: Is there an obesity paradox? *Ann. Thorac. Surg.* 2011, *91*, 42–47. [CrossRef]
12. Hartrumpf, M.; Kuehnel, R.U.; Albes, J.M. The obesity paradox is still there: A risk analysis of over 15 000 cardiosurgical patients based on body mass index. *Interact. Cardiovasc. Thorac. Surg.* 2017, *25*, 18–24. [CrossRef]
13. Mariscalco, G.; Wozniak, M.J.; Dawson, A.G.; Serraino, G.F.; Porter, R.; Nath, M.; Klersy, C.; Kumar, T.; Murphy, G.J. Body mass index and mortality among adults undergoing cardiac surgery: A nationwide study with a systematic review and meta-analysis. *Circulation* 2017, *135*, 850–863. [CrossRef] [PubMed]
14. Murphy, R.A.; Reinders, I.; Garcia, M.E.; Eiriksdottir, G.; Launer, L.J.; Benediktsson, R.; Gudnason, V.; Jonsson, P.V.; Harris, T.B. Adipose tissue, muscle, and function: Potential mediators of associations between body weight and mortality in older adults with type 2 diabetes. *Diabetes Care* 2014, *37*, 3213–3219. [CrossRef] [PubMed]
15. Jiang, X.; Xu, J.; Zhen, S.; Zhu, Y. Obesity is associated with postoperative outcomes in patients undergoing cardiac surgery: A cohort study. *BMC Anesthesiol.* 2023, *23*, 3. [CrossRef] [PubMed]
16. De Santo, L.S.; Moscariello, C.; Zebele, C. Implications of obesity in cardiac surgery: Pattern of referral, physiopathology, complications, prognosis. *J. Thorac. Dis.* 2018, *10*, 4532–4539. [CrossRef] [PubMed]
17. Karra, R.; McDermott, L.; Connelly, S.; Smith, P.; Sexton, D.J.; Kaye, K.S. Risk factors for 1-year mortality after postoperative mediastinitis. *J. Thorac. Cardiovasc. Surg.* 2006, *132*, 537–543. [CrossRef]
18. Molina, J.E.; Lew, R.S.; Hyland, K.J. Postoperative sternal dehiscence in obese patients: Incidence and prevention. *Ann. Thorac. Surg.* 2004, *78*, 912–917; discussion 912–917. [CrossRef]
19. Vargo, P.R.; Steffen, R.J.; Bakaeen, F.G.; Navale, S.; Soltesz, E.G. The impact of obesity on cardiac surgery outcomes. *J. Card. Surg.* 2018, *33*, 588–594. [CrossRef]
20. Rahmanian, P.B.; Adams, D.H.; Castillo, J.G.; Chikwe, J.; Bodian, C.A.; Filsoufi, F. Impact of body mass index on early outcome and late survival in patients undergoing coronary artery bypass grafting or valve surgery or both. *Am. J. Cardiol.* 2007, *100*, 1702–1708. [CrossRef]
21. Murtuza, B.; Pepper, J.R.; Stanbridge, R.D.; Jones, C.; Rao, C.; Darzi, A.; Athanasiou, T. Minimal access aortic valve replacement: Is it worth it? *Ann. Thorac. Surg.* 2008, *85*, 1121–1131. [CrossRef]
22. Plass, A.; Scheffel, H.; Alkadhi, H.; Kaufmann, P.; Genoni, M.; Falk, V.; Grünenfelder, J. Aortic valve replacement through a minimally invasive approach: Preoperative planning, surgical technique, and outcome. *Ann. Thorac. Surg.* 2009, *88*, 1851–1856. [CrossRef] [PubMed]
23. Wilbring, M.; Arzt, S.; Alexiou, K.; Charitos, E.; Matschke, K.; Kappert, U. Clinical Safety and Efficacy of the Transaxillary Access Route for Minimally Invasive Aortic Valve Replacement. *Thorac. Cardiovasc. Surg.* 2023, *71*, DGTHG-V47. [CrossRef]
24. Wilbring, M.; Arzt, S.; Alexiou, K.; Matschke, K.; Kappert, U. Surgery without visible scars-double valve surgery using the right lateral access. *Ann. Cardiothorac. Surg.* 2020, *9*, 424–426. [CrossRef]
25. Wilbring, M.; Matschke, K.E.; Alexiou, K.; Di Eusanio, M.; Kappert, U. Surgery without scars: Right lateral access for minimally invasive aortic valve replacement. *Thorac. Cardiovasc. Surg.* 2021, *69*, 461–465. [CrossRef]
26. Coti, I.; Haberl, T.; Scherzer, S.; Werner, P.; Shabanian, S.; Kocher, A.; Laufer, G.; Andreas, M. Outcome of rapid deployment aortic valves: Long-term experience after 700 implants. *Ann. Cardiothorac. Surg.* 2020, *9*, 314–321. [CrossRef]
27. Williams, M.L.; Flynn, C.D.; Mamo, A.A.; Tian, D.H.; Kappert, U.; Wilbring, M.; Folliguet, T.; Fiore, A.; Miceli, A.; D'Onofrio, A.; et al. Long-term outcomes of sutureless and rapid-deployment aortic valve replacement: A systematic review and meta-analysis. *Ann. Cardiothorac. Surg.* 2020, *9*, 265–279. [CrossRef]
28. Pollari, F.; Mamdooh, H.; Hitzl, W.; Grossmann, I.; Vogt, F.; Fischlein, T. Ten years' experience with the sutureless aortic valve replacement: Incidence and predictors for survival and valve durability at follow-up. *Eur. J. Cardiothorac. Surg.* 2023, *63*, ezac572. [CrossRef]
29. Rao, P.N.; Kumar, A.S. Aortic valve replacement through right thoracotomy. *Tex. Heart Inst. J.* 1993, *20*, 307–308.

30. Cosgrove, D.M., 3rd; Sabik, J.F. Minimally invasive approach for aortic valve operations. *Ann. Thorac. Surg.* **1996**, *62*, 596–597. [CrossRef]
31. Svensson, L.G.; D'Agostino, R.S. "J" incision minimal-access valve operations. *Ann. Thorac. Surg.* **1998**, *66*, 1110–1112. [CrossRef]
32. Lamelas, J. Minimally invasive aortic valve replacement: The "Miami Method". *Ann. Cardiothorac. Surg.* **2015**, *4*, 71–77. [PubMed]
33. Van Praet, K.M.; Van Kampen, A.; Kofler, M.; Unbehaun, A.; Hommel, M.; Jacobs, S.; Falk, V.; Kempfert, J. Minimally invasive surgical aortic valve replacement through a right anterolateral thoracotomy. *Multimed. Man. Cardiothorac. Surg.* **2020**, *2020*. [CrossRef]
34. Beckmann, A.; Meyer, R.; Eberhardt, J.; Gummert, J.; Falk, V. German heart surgery report 2023: The annual updated registry of the german society for thoracic and cardiovascular surgery. *Thorac. Cardiovasc. Surg.* **2024**, *72*, 329–345. [CrossRef] [PubMed]
35. Phan, K.; Xie, A.; Di Eusanio, M.; Yan, T.D. A meta-analysis of minimally invasive versus conventional sternotomy for aortic valve replacement. *Ann. Thorac. Surg.* **2014**, *98*, 1499–1511. [CrossRef]
36. Doenst, T.; Lamelas, J. Do we have enough evidence for minimally-invasive cardiac surgery? A critical review of scientific and non-scientific information. *J. Cardiovasc. Surg.* **2017**, *58*, 613–623. [CrossRef]
37. Brown, M.L.; McKellar, S.H.; Sundt, T.M.; Schaff, H.V. Ministernotomy versus conventional sternotomy for aortic valve replacement: A systematic review and meta-analysis. *J. Thorac. Cardiovasc. Surg.* **2009**, *137*, 670–679.e5. [CrossRef]
38. Scarci, M.; Young, C.; Fallouh, H. Is ministernotomy superior to conventional approach for aortic valve replacement? *Interact. Cardiovasc. Thorac. Surg.* **2009**, *9*, 314–317. [CrossRef]
39. Modi, P.; Hassan, A.; Chitwood, W.R., Jr. Minimally invasive mitral valve surgery: A systematic review and meta-analysis. *Eur. J. Cardiothorac. Surg.* **2008**, *34*, 943–952. [CrossRef]
40. Santana, O.; Reyna, J.; Grana, R.; Buendia, M.; Lamas, G.A.; Lamelas, J. Outcomes of minimally invasive valve surgery versus standard sternotomy in obese patients undergoing isolated valve surgery. *Ann. Thorac. Surg.* **2011**, *91*, 406–410. [CrossRef]
41. Abud, B.; Saydam, O.; Engin, A.Y.; Karaarslan, K.; Kunt, A.G.; Karacelik, M. Outcomes of aortic valve replacement via right anterior minithoracotomy and central cannulation versus conventional aortic valve replacement in obese patients. *Braz. J. Cardiovasc. Surg.* **2022**, *37*, 875–882. [CrossRef]
42. Xie, X.B.; Dai, X.F.; Qiu, Z.H.; Jiang, D.B.; Wu, Q.S.; Dong, Y.; Chen, L.W. Do obese patients benefit from isolated aortic valve replacement through a partial upper sternotomy? *J. Cardiothorac. Surg.* **2022**, *17*, 179. [CrossRef] [PubMed]
43. Cammertoni, F.; Bruno, P.; Pavone, N.; Nesta, M.; Chiariello, G.A.; Grandinetti, M.; D'Avino, S.; Sanesi, V.; D'Errico, D.; Massetti, M. Outcomes of minimally invasive aortic valve replacement in obese patients: A propensity-matched study. *Braz. J. Cardiovasc. Surg.* **2024**, *39*, e20230159. [CrossRef] [PubMed]
44. Pisano, C.; Totaro, P.; Triolo, O.F.; Argano, V. Advantages of minimal access versus conventional aortic valve replacement in elderly or severely obese patients. *Innovations* **2017**, *12*, 102–108. [CrossRef]
45. Welp, H.A.; Herlemann, I.; Martens, S.; Deschka, H. Outcomes of aortic valve replacement via partial upper sternotomy versus conventional aortic valve replacement in obese patients. *Interact. Cardiovasc. Thorac. Surg.* **2018**, *27*, 481–486. [CrossRef]
46. Girgis, S.W.G.; Leon, K.N.; Nekhila, W.S.B. Mini-sternotomy aortic valve replacement in morbid obesity: Can the little offer the greater? *Egypt. J. Hosp. Med.* **2022**, *89*, 7745–7748. [CrossRef]
47. Furukawa, N.; Kuss, O.; Aboud, A.; Schonbrodt, M.; Renner, A.; Hakim Meibodi, K.; Becker, T.; Zittermann, A.; Gummert, J.F.; Borgermann, J. Ministernotomy versus conventional sternotomy for aortic valve replacement: Matched propensity score analysis of 808 patients. *Eur. J. Cardiothorac. Surg.* **2014**, *46*, 221–226; discussion 226–227. [CrossRef]
48. Acharya, M.; Harling, L.; Moscarelli, M.; Ashrafian, H.; Athanasiou, T.; Casula, R. Influence of body mass index on outcomes after minimal-access aortic valve replacement through a J-shaped partial upper sternotomy. *J. Cardiothorac. Surg.* **2016**, *11*, 74. [CrossRef]
49. Lim, J.Y.; Deo, S.V.; Altarabsheh, S.E.; Jung, S.H.; Erwin, P.J.; Markowitz, A.H.; Park, S.J. Conventional versus minimally invasive aortic valve replacement: Pooled analysis of propensity-matched data. *J. Card. Surg.* **2015**, *30*, 125–134. [CrossRef]
50. Abdelaal, S.A.; Abdelrahim, N.A.; Mamdouh, M.; Ahmed, N.; Ahmed, T.R.; Hefnawy, M.T.; Alaqori, L.K.; Abozaid, M. Comparative effects of minimally invasive approaches vs. conventional for obese patients undergoing aortic valve replacement: A systematic review and network meta-analysis. *BMC Cardiovasc. Disord.* **2023**, *23*, 392. [CrossRef]
51. Wilbring, M.; Alexiou, K.; Schmidt, T.; Petrov, A.; Taghizadeh-Waghefi, A.; Charitos, E.; Matschke, K.; Arzt, S.; Kappert, U. Safety and Efficacy of the Transaxillary Access for Minimally Invasive Aortic Valve Surgery. *Medicina* **2023**, *59*, 160. [CrossRef]
52. Murphy, G.J.; Reeves, B.C.; Rogers, C.A.; Rizvi, S.I.; Culliford, L.; Angelini, G.D. Increased mortality, postoperative morbidity, and cost after red blood cell transfusion in patients having cardiac surgery. *Circulation* **2007**, *116*, 2544–2552. [CrossRef]
53. Rahmanian, P.B.; Kaya, S.; Eghbalzadeh, K.; Menghesha, H.; Madershahian, N.; Wahlers, T. Rapid deployment aortic valve replacement: Excellent results and increased effective orifice areas. *Ann. Thorac. Surg.* **2018**, *105*, 24–30. [CrossRef]

Disclaimer/Publisher's Note: The statements, opinions and data contained in all publications are solely those of the individual author(s) and contributor(s) and not of MDPI and/or the editor(s). MDPI and/or the editor(s) disclaim responsibility for any injury to people or property resulting from any ideas, methods, instructions or products referred to in the content.

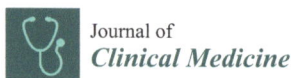

Article

Can Obesity Serve as a Barrier to Minimally Invasive Mitral Valve Surgery? Overcoming the Limitations—A Multivariate Logistic Regression Analysis

Sadeq Ali-Hasan-Al-Saegh [1,*], Florian Helms [1], Khalil Aburahma [1], Sho Takemoto [2], Nunzio Davide De Manna [1], Lukman Amanov [1], Fabio Ius [1], Jan Karsten [3], Alina Zubarevich [1], Bastian Schmack [1], Tim Kaufeld [1], Aron-Frederik Popov [1], Arjang Ruhparwar [1], Jawad Salman [1,†] and Alexander Weymann [1,†]

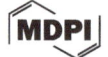

1. Department of Cardiothoracic, Transplantation and Vascular Surgery, Hannover Medical School, 30625 Hannover, Germany; ius.fabio@mh-hannover.de (F.I.)
2. Center for Transplantation Sciences, Department of Surgery, Massachusetts General Hospital and Harvard Medical School, Boston, MA 02114, USA
3. Department of Anaesthesiology and Intensive Care Medicine, Hannover Medical School, 30625 Hannover, Germany; karsten.jan@mh-hannover.de
* Correspondence: al-saegh.sadeq@mh-hannover.de; Tel.: +49-176-1532-4895
† These authors contributed equally to this work.

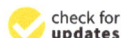

Citation: Ali-Hasan-Al-Saegh, S.; Helms, F.; Aburahma, K.; Takemoto, S.; De Manna, N.D.; Amanov, L.; Ius, F.; Karsten, J.; Zubarevich, A.; Schmack, B.; et al. Can Obesity Serve as a Barrier to Minimally Invasive Mitral Valve Surgery? Overcoming the Limitations—A Multivariate Logistic Regression Analysis. *J. Clin. Med.* **2024**, *13*, 6355. https://doi.org/10.3390/jcm13216355

Academic Editor: Manuel Wilbring

Received: 10 October 2024
Revised: 18 October 2024
Accepted: 21 October 2024
Published: 24 October 2024

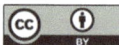

Copyright: © 2024 by the authors. Licensee MDPI, Basel, Switzerland. This article is an open access article distributed under the terms and conditions of the Creative Commons Attribution (CC BY) license (https://creativecommons.org/licenses/by/4.0/).

Abstract: Background/Objectives: Over the past two decades, significant advancements in mitral valve surgery have focused on minimally invasive techniques. Some surgeons consider obesity as a relative contraindication for minimally invasive mitral valve surgery (MIMVS). The aim of this study is to evaluate whether the specific characteristics of obese patients contribute to increased surgical complexity and whether this, in turn, leads to worse clinical outcomes compared to non-obese patients. Furthermore, we aim to explore whether these findings could substantiate the consideration of limiting this treatment option for obese patients. We investigated the outcomes of MIMVS in obese and non-obese patients at a high-volume center in Germany staffed by an experienced surgical team well-versed in perioperative management. **Methods:** A total of 934 MIMVS were performed in our high-volume center in Germany from 2011 to 2023. Of these, 196 patients had a BMI of 30 or higher (obese group), while 738 patients had a BMI below 30 (non-obese group), all of whom underwent MIMVS by right minithoracotomy. Demographic information, echocardiographic assessments, surgical data, and clinical outcome parameters were collected for all patients. **Results:** There was no significant difference in in-hospital, 30-day, and late mortality between groups (obese vs. non-obese: 6 [3.0%] vs. 14 [1.8%], $p = 0.40$; 6 [3.0%] vs. 14 [1.8%], $p = 0.40$; 13 [6.6%] vs. 39 [5.3%], $p = 0.48$, respectively). Respiratory insufficiency and arrhythmia occurred more frequently in the obese group (obese vs. non-obese: 25 [12.7%] vs. 35 [4.7%], $p < 0.001$; 35 [17.8%] vs. 77 [10.4%], $p = 0.006$). **Conclusions:** Obesity was not associated with increased early or late mortality in patients undergoing MIMVS. However, obese patients experienced higher incidences of postoperative complications, including respiratory insufficiency, arrhythmias, delirium, and wound dehiscence. Nonetheless, a multivariate logistic regression analysis indicated that obesity itself does not contraindicate MIMVS and should not be viewed as a barrier to offering this minimally invasive approach to obese patients.

Keywords: minimally invasive mitral valve surgery; mitral valve replacement; mitral valve repair; obesity; BMI

1. Introduction

Obesity has become a significant global health concern, with its prevalence continuing to rise worldwide. The global prevalence of obesity has tripled in recent decades, with around 40% of men classified as overweight (body mass index [BMI] of 25–30 kg/m^2) and 13% classified as obese (BMI > 30 kg/m^2) in 2016 [1]. Obesity is recognized as a considerable risk factor for various health conditions, including diabetes, cardiovascular disorders, and respiratory complications [2]. Given the link between obesity and multiple cardiovascular risk factors, it is likely that the number of cardiac surgery patients with obesity will increase significantly in the coming years and decades. In the context of cardiac surgery, obesity is associated with an increased likelihood of complications such as acute kidney injury and impaired wound healing, longer hospital stays, and the need for re-exploration after conventional cardiac surgeries [3–5]. The absolute prevalence of primary mitral valve regurgitation, one of the most common degenerative heart valve diseases, has significantly increased, with a 70% rise observed from 1990 to 2017 [6]. These rising trends necessitate a deeper understanding of how obesity impacts the outcomes of cardiac surgery, particularly in patients with mitral valve disease.

Over the past two decades, significant advancements in mitral valve surgery have focused on minimally invasive techniques, including minithoracotomy and robotic- and video-assisted methods. Compared to a conventional full sternotomy, minimally invasive techniques offer improved short- and mid-term outcomes, including a reduced severity of pain after surgery, shorter hospitalization, and faster recovery [7]. However, several challenges remain, particularly regarding the suitability of minimally invasive mitral valve surgery (MIMVS) for obese patients. Some surgeons consider obesity a relative contraindication for MIMVS based on several factors, such as a limited access to the mediastinum, reduced visibility associated with the increased abdominal weight elevating the right hemidiaphragm in a supine position, a higher ventilation pressure demand and risk of barotrauma, and difficulties in the management of venous drainage and arterial line pressures [8–10]. Despite these challenges, minimally invasive approaches may offer an attractive alternative for obese patients, potentially reducing the risk of complications associated with a sternotomy without compromising safety and efficacy.

The aim of this study is to evaluate whether the specific characteristics of obese patients contribute to increased surgical complexity and whether this, in turn, leads to worse clinical outcomes compared to non-obese patients. Furthermore, we aim to explore whether these findings could substantiate the consideration of limiting this treatment option for obese patients. We investigated the outcomes of MIMVS in obese and non-obese patients at a high-volume center in Germany staffed by an experienced surgical team well-versed in perioperative management. The novelty of our study, in comparison to previous studies, lies in several key aspects. First, we utilized a larger sample size of patients who underwent MIMVS through minithoracotomy, which enhances the reliability of our findings. Additionally, we conducted comprehensive follow-ups for each patient until 2024 to assess late mortality rates, providing valuable insights into long-term outcomes. Furthermore, we employed specific statistical methods, including a multivariate regression analysis, to investigate the exact impact of obesity on clinical outcomes and complications following MIMVS.

2. Materials and Methods

2.1. Study Population

From 2011 to 2023, a total of 934 MIMVS were performed in our high-volume center in Germany. Of these, 196 patients had a BMI of 30 or higher (obese group), while 738 patients had a BMI below 30 (non-obese group), all of whom underwent MIMVS by right minithoracotomy. We collected perioperative and postoperative (post-op) data from our database. The inclusion criteria encompassed all etiologies of mitral valve disease, including degenerative, ischemic, rheumatic, and infective causes. Patients with severe extracardiac arteriopathy that precluded the establishment of a cardiopulmonary bypass (CPB) through the groin vessels, as well as those with a significantly impaired left ventricular ejection fraction, were excluded from the study.

2.2. Physical Measurements

Height was measured without shoes using a standard wall-mounted stadiometer, and weight was recorded using calibrated physician-grade scales. Trained personnel conducted these measurements to ensure accuracy. Body mass index (BMI) was calculated using the standard formula: BMI = weight (kg)/height (m)^2.

2.3. Ethical Statement

In accordance with local German protocols, study approval by the institutional ethical review board was waived given the retrospective and non-interventional design of this study.

2.4. Surgical Technique

The surgical techniques, including the right minithoracotomy approach, as well as the perfusion strategies and aortic clamping techniques employed in this study, have been previously described by our team [11]. All surgeries were conducted through a right minithoracotomy, with continuous carbon dioxide insufflation maintained throughout the procedure. In brief, a cardiopulmonary bypass (CPB) was typically initiated via the right femoral vessels, and single-lung ventilation was utilized. Initially, a two-stage venous cannula was placed into the superior vena cava using echocardiographic guidance, followed by the insertion of an arterial cannula. The pericardium was incised 3 to 4 cm above the phrenic nerve. Unfractionated heparin was administered intravenously to achieve an activated clotting time exceeding 450 s, which was fully reversed with protamine after removal of the venous cannula.

2.5. Follow-Up and Patient Data Collection

All patients were followed up for 30 days after surgery, and their survival was tracked until August 2024. Demographic information, echocardiographic assessments, surgical data, and clinical outcome parameters were collected for all patients. This included the incidence of post-op complications such as wound dehiscence, arrhythmia, right ventricular failure, new-onset atrial fibrillation (NOAF), new myocardial infarction, the need for pacemaker implantation, thromboembolic events, respiratory insufficiency, the necessity for cardiopulmonary resuscitation, acute renal failure requiring dialysis, ischemic stroke, delirium, intracranial hemorrhage, major bleeding necessitating re-thoracotomy, and sepsis. Additional metrics included intubation duration, duration of catecholamine therapy, and transfusion of blood cells or products. Post-op early mortality was defined as death occurring during the hospital stay or within the first 30 days after surgery, while late mortality referred to deaths occurring beyond 30 days.

2.6. Echocardiographic Assessment

Transthoracic echocardiography was routinely performed both before surgery and prior to discharge. The echocardiographic parameters collected included left ventricular ejection fraction (LVEF), grades of mitral valve insufficiency (MI) II, III, and IV, and grades of mitral valve stenosis (MS) II and III.

2.7. Statistical Analysis

Data analysis was performed using SPSS version 28.01.1. Continuous variables were summarized as the mean with standard deviation (SD), while categorical variables were reported as counts and percentages relative to the total sample size. A Mann–Whitney U test was utilized to compare continuous variables, whereas a Chi-square test was used for categorical comparisons. A Fisher's exact test was conducted when any cell in the cross-tabulation had an expected count of less than 5. Multivariate logistic regression models were fitted for each dichotomous outcome, while multivariate linear regression models were used for continuous outcome variables. A multivariate logistic regression analysis was selected for this study as it facilitates the prediction of a binary outcome, such as the occurrence or non-occurrence of postoperative complications, by considering multiple independent variables, including obesity and various patient characteristics. Results from the regression analysis were reported as odds ratios (OR) along with 95% confidence intervals (CIs). Each regression model was conducted independently. A p-value of less than 0.05 was considered statistically significant.

3. Results

3.1. Patient Demographics and Perioperative and Procedure Characteristics

Of the 934 patients who underwent MIMVS, 196 patients (21.0%) had a BMI $\geq$ 30 kg/m^2, and 738 patients (79.0%) had a BMI < 30 kg/m^2 (Figure 1). Patient demographics and pre-and intraoperative data are summarized in Tables 1 and 2. Male gender (obese: 99 [50.5%] vs. non-obese: 411 [55.6%], p = 0.02), insulin-dependent diabetes mellitus (obese: 18 [9.1%] vs. non-obese: 18 [2.4%], p < 0.001), pulmonary hypertension (obese: 104 [53.0%] vs. non-obese: 309 [41.8%], p = 0.03), arterial hypertension (obese: 167 [85.2%] vs. non-obese: 460 [62.3%], p < 0.001), hyperlipidemia (obese: 118 [60.2%] vs. non-obese: 304 [22.4%], p < 0.001), atrial fibrillation (obese: 111 [56.6%] vs. non-obese: 313 [42.34], p < 0.001), mitral valve stenosis (obese: 23 [11.7%] vs. non-obese: 34 [4.6%], p < 0.001), mitral valve prolapse (obese: 83 [42.3%] vs. non-obese: 461 [62.4%], p < 0.001), endocarditis (obese: 8 [4.0%] vs. non-obese: 67 [9.0%], p = 0.02), and maximum mitral valve gradient (obese: 10.1 $\pm$ 5.2 vs. non-obese: 8.9 $\pm$ 5.1 mmHg, p = 0.007) were significantly different between groups. Mechanical mitral valve replacement was performed more frequently in the obese group (obese: 35 [17.8%] vs. non-obese: 73 [9.8%], p = 0.004), and mitral valve repair was performed more frequently in the non-obese group (obese: 102 [52.0%] vs. non-obese: 479 [64.9%], p < 0.001). Among mitral valve repair, neochordae was utilized more frequently in the non-obese group (obese: 61 [31.1%] vs. non-obese: 343 [46.4%], p < 0.001). The obese group needed a significantly longer duration of surgery (obese: 224.1 $\pm$ 65.7 vs. non-obese: 210.8 $\pm$ 54.5 [46.4%], p < 0.001). All other demographics were not significantly different between groups.

Table 1. Demographics and preoperative data.

Variables	Non-Obese Group (N = 738)	Obese Group (N = 196)	p-Value
Age	64.5 $\pm$ 13.9	66.4 $\pm$ 11.0	0.08
Elderly cases (over 75 years of age)	196 (26.5%)	50 (25.5%)	0.43
Male Gender	411 (55.6%)	99 (50.5)	0.02 *
Elective operations	492 (66.6%)	122 (62.2%)	
Urgent operations	196 (26.5%)	64 (32.6%)	0.19
Emergency operations	50 (6.7%)	10 (5.1%)	
Peripheral artery disease	53 (7.1%)	17 (8.6%)	0.28
COPD	106 (14.3%)	35 (17.8%)	0.13
Active endocarditis	56 (7.5%)	8 (4%)	0.07
Insulin-dependent diabetes mellitus	18 (2.4%)	18 (9.1%)	0.001 *
Recent myocardial infarction	8 (1.0%)	5 (2.5%)	0.11
Preoperative stroke	58 (7.8%)	16 (8.1%)	0.49
Neurological symptoms	74 (10.0%)	23 (11.7%)	0.51
Pulmonary hypertension	309 (41.8%)	104 (53.0%)	0.03 *
Coronary artery disease	199 (26.9%)	64 (32.6%)	0.12
Smoking history	153 (20.7%)	49 (25%)	0.20
Arterial hypertension	460 (62.3%)	167 (85.2%)	0.001 *
Hyperlipidemia	304 (22.4%)	118 (60.2%)	0.001 *
Atrial fibrillation	313 (42.4%)	111 (56.6%)	0.001 *
Mitral valve stenosis	34 (4.6%)	23 (11.7%)	0.001 *
Mitral valve regurgitation	642 (86.9%)	168 (85.7%)	0.63
Mitral valve prolapse	461(62.4%)	83 (42.3%)	0.001 *
Endocarditis	67 (9.0%)	8 (4.0%)	0.02 *
Anulus dilatation	367 (49.7%)	82 (41.8%)	0.64

Table 1. *Cont.*

Variables	Non-Obese Group (N = 738)	Obese Group (N = 196)	*p*-Value
Cardiac myxoma	8 (1.0%)	1 (0.5%)	0.87
Mean mitral valve gradient	4 ± 3.5	4.4 ± 2.2	0.25
Maximal mitral valve gradient	8.9 ± 5.1	10.1 ± 5.2	0.007 *

NYHA: New York Heart Association; COPD: chronic obstructive pulmonary disease. * *p*-value significant.

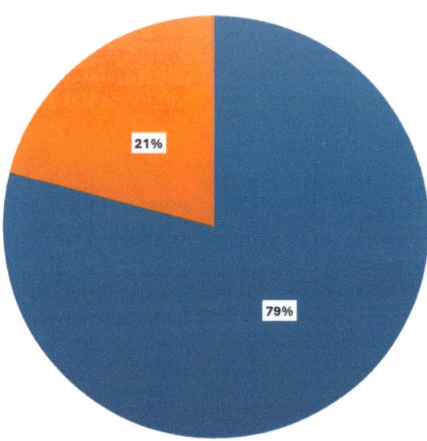

Figure 1. Distribution of patients according to obesity (BMI ≥ 30) and non-obesity (BMI < 30).

Table 2. Procedure characteristics.

Variables	Non-Obese Group (N = 738)	Obese Group (N = 196)	*p*-Value
Biological mitral valve replacement	186 (25.2%)	59 (30.1%)	0.17
Mechanical mitral valve replacement	73 (9.8%)	35 (17.8%)	0.004 *
Mitral valve repair	479 (64.9%)	102 (52.0%)	0.001 *
Plasty with neochordae	343 (46.4%)	61 (31.1%)	0.001
Cleft closure	76 (10.2%)	12 (6.1%)	0.09
Segment resection	38 (5.1%)	4 (2.0%)	0.07
Sliding plasty	8 (1.0%)	1 (0.5%)	0.69
Augmentation	27 (3.6%)	7 (3.5%)	1.0
Maze procedure	133 (18.0%)	40 (20.4%)	0.46
Duration of surgery (minutes)	210.8 ± 54.5	224.1 ± 65.7	0.004 *
Time on CPB (minutes)	78.4 ± 35.3	74.8 ± 39.5	0.21

CPB: cardiopulmonary bypass. * *p*-value significant.

3.2. Postoperative Outcomes and Echocardiographic Data

Post-op outcomes are shown in Table 3. There was no significant difference in in-hospital, 30-day, and late mortality between groups (obese vs. non-obese: 6 [3.0%] vs. 14 [1.8%], p = 0.40; 6 [3.0%] vs. 14 [1.8%], p = 0.40; 13 [6.6%] vs. 39 [5.3%], p = 0.48, respectively). Respiratory insufficiency and arrhythmia occurred more frequently in the obese group (obese vs. non-obese: 25 [12.7%] vs. non-obese: 35 [4.7%], p < 0.001; 35 [17.8%] vs. non-obese: 77 [10.4%], p = 0.006), and the incidence of new-onset atrial fibrillation (NOAF), stroke, and wound dehiscence were near significant in two groups (obese vs. non-obese: 26 [13.2%] vs. 66 [8.9%], p = 0.07; 7 [3.5%] vs. 11 [1.4%], p = 0.07; 19 [9.6%] vs. 42 [5.6%], p = 0.06, respectively). The incidence of delirium was higher in the obese group (obese: 11 [5.6%] vs. non-obese: 18 [2.4%], p = 0.003) (Figure 2). There was no significant difference in other variables.

Table 3. Postoperative data.

Variables	Non-Obese Group (N = 738)	Obese Group (N = 196)	p-Value
In-hospital mortality	14 (1.8%)	6 (3.0%)	0.40 [§]
30-day mortality	14 (1.8%)	6 (3.0%)	0.40 [§]
Late mortality	39 (5.3%)	13 (6.6%)	0.48
Duration of therapy with catecholamine	35.5 ± 88.5	47.5 ± 116.9	0.11
Duration of intubation (hours)	27.9 ± 97.0	47.5 ± 116.9	0.06
Erythrocyte transfusion	3.4 ± 5.1	4.1 ± 8.4	0.45
FFP transfusion	1.9 ± 4.7	1.8 ± 6.9	0.89
Platelet transfusion	0.5 ± 1.7	0.6 ± 1.3	0.75
Respiratory insufficiency	35 (4.7%)	25 (12.7%)	0.001 *[§]
Mitral valve re-operation	11 (1.4%)	2 (1.0%)	1.0
Arrhythmia	77 (10.4%)	35 (17.8%)	0.006 *[§]
ECMO/right ventricular failure	23 (3.1%)	7 (3.5%)	0.81
Re-thoracotomy	53 (7.1%)	16 (8.1%)	0.64
Major bleeding	49 (6.6%)	19 (9.6%)	0.16
New onset atrial fibrillation	66 (8.9%)	26 (13.2%)	0.07
Renal failure with new onset dialysis	23 (3.1%)	7 (3.5%)	0.81
Stroke	11 (1.4%)	7 (3.5%)	0.07
Cerebral bleeding	2 (0.3%)	2 (1.0%)	0.19
Seizure	9 (1.2%)	4 (2.0%)	0.48
Delirium	18 (2.4%)	11 (5.6%)	0.03 *[§]
Thromboembolic events	4 (0.5%)	1 (0.5%)	1.0
Wound dehiscence	42 (5.6%)	19 (9.6%)	0.06 *[§]
Sepsis	12 (1.6%)	3 (1.5%)	1.0
Myocardial infarction	2 (0.2%)	0 (0%)	1.0
Pacemaker implantation	38 (5.1%)	16 (8.1%)	0.12
CPR	13 (1.7%)	4 (2.0%)	0.76

CPB: cardiopulmonary bypass; CPR: cardiopulmonary resuscitation; ECMO: extracorporeal membrane oxygenation; FFP: fresh frozen plasma. * p-value significant. [§] Need to clarify through a multivariate regression analysis.

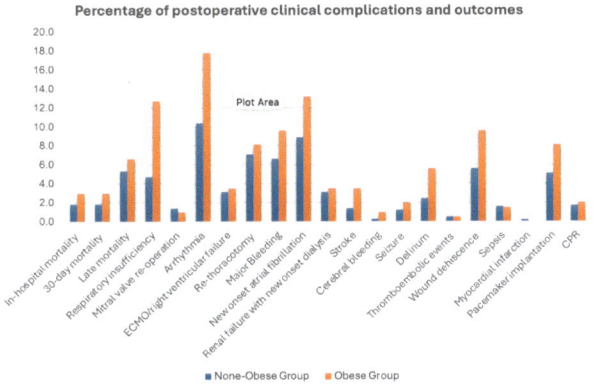

Figure 2. Percentage of postoperative clinical complications and outcomes.

Echocardiographic outcomes are displayed in Table 4. Although the non-obese group showed significantly higher preoperative (pre-op) LVEF, post-op LVEF was comparable among groups (obese vs. non-obese: 50.7 ± 18.6 vs. 55.0 ±16.3%, p = 0.002; 51.1 ± 13.3 vs. 52.0 ± 11.2%, p = 0.37). Grade II mitral stenosis (MS) was observed more frequently in the obese group preoperatively (obese: 8 [4.0%] vs. non-obese: 8 [1.0%], p = 0.007). Post-op echocardiography revealed a near-significant higher incidence of grade I MI in the non-obese group (obese: 27 [13.7%] vs. non-obese: 148 [20.0%], p = 0.07), while grade II or higher MI and MS were rarely observed in both groups.

Table 4. Echocardiographic assessments.

Time	Variables	Non-Obese Group (N = 738)	Obese Group (N = 196)	p-Value
Preoperative	LVEF	55 ± 16.3	50.7 ± 18.6	0.002 *
	MI II	115 (15.5%)	57 (29.0%)	0.07
	MI III	475 (64.3%)	123 (62.7%)	0.70
	MI IV	71 (9.6%)	10 (5.1%)	0.79
	MS II	8 (1.0%)	8 (4.0%)	0.007 *
	MS III	17 (2.3%)	9 (4.5%)	0.07
Postoperative	LVEF	52 ± 11.2	51.1 ± 13.3	0.37
	MI I	148 (20.0%)	27 (13.7%)	0.07
	MI II	19 (2.5%)	2 (1.0%)	0.27
	MI III	0 (0%)	0 (0%)	-
	MI IV	0 (0%)	0 (0%)	-
	MS II	1 (0.1%)	0 (0%)	1.0
	MS III	1 (0.1%)	0 (0%)	1.0

LVEF: left ventricular ejection fraction; MI: mitral valve insufficiency; MS: mitral valve stenosis; Pre-OP: preoperative; Post-OP: postoperative. * p-value significant.

3.3. Regression Model: Impact of Obesity on Mortality and Postoperative Outcomes

- *Mortality*

Obesity was not significant for in-hospital and 30-day mortality in the multivariate logistic regression analysis (odds ratio (OR): 3.82, 95% CI: [0.15–92.27], p = 0.4; OR: 1.61, 95% CI: [0.12–20.36], p = 0.71, respectively) (Table 5). No other pre-op conditions or procedural characteristics were not a risk factor for mortality.

- *Arrhythmia*

Obesity was not an independent predictive factor for post-op arrhythmia (OR: 1.18, 95% CI: [0.68–2.06], p = 0.54). Both mechanical MV replacement and MV repair were protective factors (OR: 0.23, 95% CI: [0.08–0.64], p < 0.001; OR: 0.47, 95% CI: [0.26–0.85], p = 0.01, respectively). Pre-op AF was a substantial risk of post-op arrhythmia (OR: 3.23, 95% CI: [1.91–5.48], p < 0.001).

- *Respiratory insufficiency*

Obesity did not increase the risk of post-op respiratory insufficiency (OR 0.96, 95% CI 0.44–2.10, p = 0.93). Pre-op LVEF was associated with the risk of post-op respiratory failure (OR 0.97, 95% CI 0.96–0.99, p = 0.01), whereas pre-op pulmonary hypertension showed borderline significance as a predictive factor (OR 2.01, 95% CI 0.98–4.09, p = 0.05).

- *Wound dehiscence and delirium*

Our logistic regression analysis revealed obesity was not a risk factor for either wound dehiscence or delirium (OR: 1.71, 95% CI: [0.885–3.336], p = 0.11; OR: 1.03, 95%

CI: [0.34–3.13], $p = 0.95$, respectively). Furthermore, no significant independent predictive factors were identified for either wound dehiscence or delirium.

Table 5. Multivariate logistic regression analysis.

Variables	OR	Lower–Upper 95% CI		p-value
Intrahospital Mortality				
Obesity	3.82	0.15	92.27	0.40
Pulmonary HTN	0.85	0.04	15.92	0.91
Arterial HTN	14.76	0.00	-	0.99
HLP	44.87	0.00	-	0.99
Pre-OP AF	0.77	0.03	15.11	0.86
Mitral valve stenosis	0.00	0.00	-	0.99
Endocarditis	0.00	0.00	-	0.99
Gender	76.63	0.00	-	0.99
IDDM	0.00	0.00	-	0.99
Mitral valve prolapse	1.47	0.06	36.58	0.81
Mechanical MVR	0.00	0.00	-	0.99
Mitral valve repair	0.67	0.02	18.20	0.81
Pre-OP LVEF	1.04	0.90	1.19	0.57
Maximal gradient	1.02	0.67	1.54	0.91
30-Day Mortality				
Obesity	1.61	0.12	20.36	0.71
Pulmonary HTN	1.53	0.12	19.06	0.73
Arterial HTN	5.00	0.00	-	0.99
HLP	1.42	0.11	17.18	0.78
Pre-OP AF	1.46	0.11	18.50	0.76
Mitral valve stenosis	0.00	0.00	-	0.99
Endocarditis	0.00	0.00	-	0.99
Gender	2.07	0.18	22.92	0.55
IDDM	0.00	0.00	-	0.99
Mitral valve prolapse	0.51	0.03	7.95	0.63
Mechanical MVR	0.00	0.00	-	0.99
Mitral valve repair	0.24	0.01	3.66	0.30
Pre-OP LVEF	1.01	0.93	1.11	0.70
Maximal gradient	0.92	0.72	1.18	0.53
Wound Dehiscence				
Obesity	1.71	0.885	3.336	0.11
Pulmonary HTN	1.00	0.552	1.838	0.98
Arterial HTN	1.30	0.649	2.613	0.45
HLP	0.73	0.39	1.35	0.32
Pre-OP AF	1.62	0.87	2.99	0.12
Mitral valve stenosis	0.59	0.15	2.32	0.45
Endocarditis	0.87	0.24	3.14	0.83
Gender	0.77	0.43	1.37	0.38
IDDM	2.35	0.80	6.86	0.11
Mitral valve prolapse	0.78	0.38	1.59	0.51

Table 5. *Cont.*

	Wound Dehiscence			
Variables	OR	Lower–Upper 95% CI		p-value
Mechanical MVR	2.34	0.91	6.02	0.07
Mitral valve repair	1.15	0.50	2.63	0.73
Pre-OP LVEF	1.00	0.98	1.02	0.90
Maximal gradient	0.95	0.89	1.02	0.20
	Arrhythmia			
Variables	OR	Lower–Upper 95% CI		p-value
Obesity	1.18	0.68	2.06	0.54
Pulmonary HTN	0.93	0.58	1.51	0.79
Arterial HTN	1.54	0.862	2.75	0.14
HLP	0.88	0.54	1.42	0.60
Pre-OP AF	3.23	1.91	5.48	0.001
Mitral valve stenosis	0.73	0.27	1.97	0.53
Endocarditis	0.00	0.00	-	0.99
Gender	0.96	0.61	1.53	0.89
IDDM	1.50	0.54	4.19	0.43
Mitral valve prolapse	0.84	0.48	1.46	0.54
Mechanical MVR	0.23	0.08	0.64	0.001
Mitral valve repair	0.47	0.26	0.85	0.01
Pre-OP LVEF	1.00	0.99	1.02	0.29
Maximal gradient	1.02	0.97	1.07	0.34
	Delirium			
Variables	OR	Lower–Upper 95% CI		p-value
Obesity	1.03	0.34	3.13	0.95
Pulmonary HTN	1.39	0.53	3.64	0.49
Arterial HTN	0.92	0.30	2.75	0.88
HLP	2.94	0.99	8.73	0.05
Pre-OP AF	2.34	0.83	6.60	0.10
Mitral valve stenosis	0.00	0.00	-	0.99
Endocarditis	1.30	0.15	10.87	0.80
Gender	1.28	0.50	3.26	0.59
IDDM	1.19	0.14	10.07	0.86
Mitral valve prolapse	1.49	0.50	4.43	0.47
Mechanical MVR	0.41	0.04	3.56	0.42
Mitral valve repair	0.80	0.25	2.53	0.71
Pre-OP LVEF	0.99	0.96	1.02	0.80
Maximal gradient	1.03	0.92	1.14	0.59
	Respiratory Insufficiency			
Variables	OR	Lower–Upper 95% CI		p-value
Obesity	0.96	0.44	2.10	0.93
Pulmonary HTN	2.01	0.98	4.09	0.05
Arterial HTN	1.79	0.74	4.31	0.19
HLP	1.89	0.91	3.92	0.08
Pre-OP AF	1.37	0.68	2.77	0.37
Mitral valve stenosis	0.54	0.11	2.57	0.44

Table 5. *Cont.*

	Respiratory Insufficiency		
Variables	OR	Lower–Upper 95% CI	*p*-value
Endocarditis	0.83	0.17 3.93	0.81
Gender	0.85	0.43 1.68	0.64
IDDM	0.79	0.17 3.70	0.77
Mitral valve prolapse	0.94	0.42 2.07	0.88
Mechanical MVR	0.96	0.34 2.73	0.95
Mitral valve repair	0.75	0.32 1.74	0.51
Pre-OP LVEF	0.97	0.96 0.99	0.01
Maximal gradient	1.03	0.96 1.10	0.32

AF, atrial fibrillation; CI, confidence interval; HLP, hyperlipidemia; HTN, hypertension; IDDM, insulin-dependent diabetes mellitus; LVEF, left ventricular ejection fraction; MVR, mitral valve replacement; OR, odds ratio; Pre-OP, preoperative; Post-OP, postoperative.

4. Discussion

Our study revealed that obesity did not contribute to an increased risk of either early or late mortality for patients who underwent MIMVS. Although respiratory insufficiency, arrhythmia, delirium, and wound dehiscence were observed more frequently in the obese group, obesity was not identified as an independent factor for these postoperative morbidities. Notably, despite both groups having a comparable mean patient age, mechanical MV replacement was more frequently performed in the obese group. In contrast, MV repair was more common in the non-obese group. Additionally, the obese group had significantly longer operative times, and a higher incidence of grade II MS was observed in postoperative echocardiography. While these findings suggest that the complexity of surgery may increase in obese patients, leading to a higher risk of certain complications, obesity alone does not appear to contraindicate MIMVS.

Obesity has emerged as a major global health issue, with prevalence rates continuing to rise globally, including across Europe. The World Health Organization (WHO) reported that the global obesity rate has almost doubled since 1980, and nearly 60% of adults in the European region are classified as overweight (BMI $\geq$ 25 kg/m^2) or obese (BMI $\geq$ 30 kg/m^2) [12]. The age group with the highest prevalence is those between 65 and 74 years old [12]. In Germany, the obesity rate stands at 19%, with similar rates observed between men and women [13].

Studies consistently have shown that obesity is associated with a higher risk of prolonged mechanical ventilation, pneumonia, deep sternal wound infections, acute renal failure, post-op AF, increased medical costs, and extended ICU/hospital stays in patients undergoing cardiac surgery [4,14,15]. While some large population studies have found no association between obesity and increased mortality [4,14] including in patients with morbid obesity (BMI $\geq$ 40 kg/m^2) [14], other studies have reported a higher mortality risk in obese patients [15]. However, neither obesity nor morbid obesity has been linked to an increased mortality in patients undergoing minimally invasive cardiac surgery, including MIMVS or robotic procedures, which is consistent with our findings [8,16,17].

Mariscalco et al., using data from the UK national registry and a meta-analysis, reported that obesity (BMI 30–40) was associated with lower mortality, while underweight patients exhibited increased mortality after cardiac surgery compared to those with normal weight [17]. Even after adjusting for confounding factors in a multivariate analysis, mortality was found to be 15–20% lower in the obese population [17]. Contrary to the expectation that obese patients would be at higher risk, this phenomenon of lower mortality in obese patients has been observed in several studies and is known as the "obesity paradox" [18]. This paradox has been documented not only in cardiac surgery outcomes but also in conditions such as heart failure, chronic obstructive lung disease, cancer, and chronic kidney disease [19]. Mariscalco and colleagues further suggested that the observed reduction in mortality among obese patients might challenge the conventional practice of advising preoperative weight loss in this population [17]. However, Carnethon et al. have pointed out the limitations of observational studies, emphasizing the potential for selection bias and the challenges of establishing causal relationships in such research designs [20]. While there may be short-term benefits for obese patients undergoing cardiac surgery, the long-term impact of obesity remains uncertain. Obese patients have higher risks for deep sternal wound infections and dialysis, both of which could adversely affect long-term outcomes [17]. Minimally invasive cardiac surgery offers the advantage of avoiding sternotomy, which can mitigate the risk of deep sternal wound infections. Additionally, in our study, there was no significant difference in the incidence of dialysis-requiring renal failure between obese and non-obese patients. These results suggest that obese patients may benefit from a minimally invasive approach by potentially avoiding these serious complications, highlighting the advantages of this approach for managing obese patients undergoing cardiac surgery.

Although mortality rates between obese and non-obese patients undergoing MIMVS have been shown to be comparable, obesity has been associated with an increased risk of complications, even in minimally invasive cardiac surgery [8,21,22]. These complications include a higher incidence of arrhythmias, surgical site infections, prolonged ventilation times, and extended hospital stays. Similarly, in our analysis, the obese group had a significantly higher incidence of respiratory insufficiency, arrhythmia, delirium, and wound dehiscence. On the other hand, Kitahara et al. reported no significant differences in morbidity between obese and non-obese patients undergoing robotic coronary artery bypass grafting [16]. However, it is important to note that approximately 60% of these procedures were total endoscopic in nature, with minimal incisions, and the use of CPB was limited to around 30% [16].

The pathophysiology of obesity-related complications in cardiac surgery is multifaceted. Impaired wound healing in obese patients can be attributed to poor vascularity and the tenuous structure of adipose tissue, leading to relative vascular insufficiency and decreased oxygen tension [23]. This may result in reduced collagen synthesis, impaired infection resistance, and compromised wound healing processes [23]. These factors may explain the increased wound healing disturbances in obese patients undergoing MIMVS, despite the smaller incisions compared to median sternotomy. Obesity also increases the risk of postoperative arrhythmias, particularly atrial fibrillation, due to excess adipose tissue altering atrial electrophysiology and obesity-associated atrial dilation [24]. Additionally, obesity leads to reduced lung capacity, functional residual volume, and shallow, fast breathing, potentially explaining the higher incidence of postoperative respiratory failure [25]. Interestingly, some observational studies report an "obesity paradox" for postoperative delirium, suggesting that a higher body weight may have a protective effect [26]. However, advanced age remains a significant risk factor for postoperative delirium, even within obese patient populations [27]. In our cohort, the obese group had a statistically near-significant higher age, which may have contributed to the higher incidence of delirium. Nevertheless, the mechanisms linking obesity and postoperative delirium remain unclear, warranting further investigation.

Santana et al. reported lower morbidity and mortality, including reduced incidences of renal failure, deep wound infections, blood transfusion, and shorter ICU and hospital stays, in patients who underwent a minimally invasive approach for isolated valve lesions compared to a median sternotomy [28]. However, aortic cross-clamp and CPB times were significantly longer in the minimally invasive group, suggesting that this approach may present greater technical challenges in obese patients compared to those with a normal body weight [28]. In our study, CPB times were similar between the groups; however, the overall duration of surgery was longer in the obese group, and MV replacement was more frequently performed than MV repair. Additionally, postoperative grade II MS was observed more often in obese patients. These findings indicate that specific technical difficulties associated with obesity may influence procedural choices, but it is also important to mention that the obese group had a significantly higher proportion of patients with MS, for whom valve replacement was the only viable option. Hadaya et al. reported that despite increased procedural complexity, high-volume centers demonstrated an independent association between greater operative volume and reduced hospitalization costs and mortality following elective cardiac operations [29]. Even though obesity itself may not be an independent risk factor for increased mortality or complications, it is evident that the technical and postoperative management challenges associated with obesity require special considerations. Therefore, such procedures should be concentrated at experienced high-volume centers where these challenges can be more effectively managed.

The clinical implications of our findings are noteworthy for the management of obese patients undergoing MIMVS. Although obesity was not found to increase early or late mortality, the higher incidence of postoperative complications highlights the need for careful perioperative planning and monitoring for this patient population. Given the technical challenges associated with obesity, surgical teams should be aware of these factors when making procedural decisions. Importantly, obesity should not be considered a contraindication for MIMVS. Our study has several limitations. First, the retrospective design inherently introduces the possibility of selection bias. Second, although we attempted to adjust for confounding variables, unmeasured factors may have influenced the outcomes, particularly regarding comorbidities and patient characteristics not captured in the dataset. Third, the study was conducted at a single center, which may limit the applicability of these findings to other institutions with lower surgical volumes. Our study presents several strengths that significantly enhance its impact. First, it utilizes a larger sample size compared to other studies, which improves the statistical power and reliability of our findings. Furthermore, the comprehensive long-term follow-up enables a thorough examination of late mortality rates. Additionally, we employed robust statistical methods, including a multivariate regression analysis, to effectively control for confounding variables, facilitating a precise assessment of how obesity influences clinical outcomes and complications.

5. Conclusions

In this study, we found that obesity was not associated with increased early or late mortality in patients undergoing MIMVS. However, obese patients experienced higher incidences of postoperative complications, including respiratory insufficiency, arrhythmias, delirium, and wound dehiscence. The complexity of the surgical procedure, reflected in longer operative times and more frequent valve replacements, suggests that obesity presents technical challenges that may influence procedural choices. Nonetheless, obesity itself does not contraindicate MIMVS and should not be viewed as a barrier to offering this minimally invasive approach to obese patients, provided that a well-experienced surgical team and perioperative management are ensured. These findings emphasize the importance of careful perioperative management and suggest that concentrating such procedures in high-volume centers with experienced teams may help optimize outcomes for obese patients. Future studies should focus on examining the long-term effects of obesity on clinical outcomes following MIMVS. Specifically, investigating aspects such as quality of life, functional status, and returning to work after MIMVS will provide valuable insights into the overall impact of obesity on recovery and patient well-being.

Author Contributions: All authors contributed to the collection of data, manuscript development, and final approval. Conceptualization, J.S., A.W. and S.A.-H.-A.-S.; methodology, S.A.-H.-A.-S., K.A., N.D.D.M., L.A., S.T. and F.I.; software, S.A.-H.-A.-S., K.A., N.D.D.M., F.H. and A.Z.; formal analysis, J.S., S.A.-H.-A.-S., J.K., F.H. and N.D.D.M.; validation, J.S., A.W., T.K., A.-F.P. and B.S.; investigation, J.S., S.A.-H.-A.-S., K.A., N.D.D.M., L.A., F.H., F.I., J.K. and A.Z.; writing—original draft preparation, S.A.-H.-A.-S., S.T., J.S. and A.W.; funding; T.K. and A.R.; writing—review and editing, A.W., J.S., S.A.-H.-A.-S., S.T., A.Z. and B.S.; supervision, J.S., A.-F.P., A.W., B.S. and A.R. All authors have read and agreed to the published version of the manuscript.

Funding: This research received no external funding.

Institutional Review Board Statement: Ethical review and approval were waived for this study due to its retrospective and non-interventional design.

Informed Consent Statement: This study was conducted in accordance with the Declaration of Helsinki. Ethical approval was granted by the Medical School of Hannover's Institutional Review Board. Informed written consent was obtained from all participants, guaranteeing the confidentiality and anonymity of their data throughout the analysis.

Data Availability Statement: Data are contained within the article.

Conflicts of Interest: The authors declare no conflicts of interest.

References

1. Chooi, Y.C.; Ding, C.; Magkos, F. The epidemiology of obesity. *Metabolism* **2019**, *92*, 6–10. [CrossRef] [PubMed]
2. Poirier, P.; Giles, T.D.; Bray, G.A.; Hong, Y.; Stern, J.S.; Pi-Sunyer, F.X.; Eckel, R.H. Obesity and Cardiovascular Disease: Pathophysiology, Evaluation, and Effect of Weight Loss: An Update of the 1997 American Heart Association Scientific Statement on Obesity and Heart Disease From the Obesity Committee of the Council on Nutrition, Physical Activity, and Metabolism. *Circulation* **2006**, *113*, 898–918. [CrossRef] [PubMed]
3. Shi, N.; Liu, K.; Fan, Y.; Yang, L.; Zhang, S.; Li, X.; Wu, H.; Li, M.; Mao, H.; Xu, X.; et al. The Association between Obesity and Risk of Acute Kidney Injury after Cardiac Surgery. *Front. Endocrinol.* **2020**, *11*, 534294. [CrossRef]
4. Ghanta, R.K.; LaPar, D.J.; Zhang, Q.; Devarkonda, V.; Isbell, J.M.; Yarboro, L.T.; Kern, J.A.; Kron, I.L.; Speir, A.M.; Fonner, C.E.; et al. Obesity Increases Risk-Adjusted Morbidity, Mortality, and Cost Following Cardiac Surgery. *JAHA* **2017**, *6*, e003831. [CrossRef]
5. De Santo, L.S.; Moscariello, C.; Zebele, C. Implications of obesity in cardiac surgery: Pattern of referral, physiopathology, complications, prognosis. *J. Thorac. Dis.* **2018**, *10*, 4532–4539. [CrossRef]
6. Santangelo, G.; Bursi, F.; Faggiano, A.; Moscardelli, S.; Simeoli, P.S.; Guazzi, M.; Lorusso, R.; Carugo, S.; Faggiano, P. The Global Burden of Valvular Heart Disease: From Clinical Epidemiology to Management. *J. Clin. Med.* **2023**, *12*, 2178. [CrossRef]
7. Eqbal, A.J.; Gupta, S.; Basha, A.; Qiu, Y.; Wu, N.; Rega, F.; Chu, F.V.; Belley-Cote, E.P.; Whitlock, R.P. Minimally invasive mitral valve surgery versus conventional sternotomy mitral valve surgery: A systematic review and meta-analysis of 119 studies. *J. Card. Surg.* **2022**, *37*, 1319–1327. [CrossRef]
8. Aljanadi, F.; Toolan, C.; Theologou, T.; Shaw, M.; Palmer, K.; Modi, P. Is obesity associated with poorer outcomes in patients undergoing minimally invasive mitral valve surgery? *Eur. J. Cardio-Thorac. Surg.* **2021**, *59*, 187–191. [CrossRef]
9. Øberg, B.; Poulsen, T.D. Obesity: An anaesthetic challenge. *Acta Anaesthesiol. Scand.* **1996**, *40*, 191–200. [CrossRef]
10. Gammie, J.S.; Bartlett, S.T.; Griffith, B.P. Small-incision mitral valve repair: Safe, durable, and approaching perfection. *Ann. Surg.* **2009**, *250*, 409–415. [CrossRef]
11. Minimally Invasive Mitral Valve Surgery in Re-Do Cases—The New Standard Procedure?—PubMed. Available online: https://pubmed.ncbi.nlm.nih.gov/29490388/ (accessed on 8 October 2024).
12. WHO Regional Office for Europe. WHO European Reginal Obesity Report. 2022. Available online: https://www.who.int/europe/publications/i/item/9789289057738 (accessed on 8 October 2024).
13. Schienkiewitz, A.; Kuhnert, R.; Blume, M.; Mensink, G.B.M. Overweight and obesity among adults in Germany—Results from GEDA 2019/2020-EHIS. *J. Health Monit.* **2022**, *7*, 21–28. [CrossRef] [PubMed]
14. Wigfield, C.H.; Lindsey, J.D.; Muñoz, A.; Chopra, P.S.; Edwards, N.M.; Love, R.B. Is extreme obesity a risk factor for cardiac surgery? An analysis of patients with a BMI ≥ 40. *Eur. J. Cardio-Thorac. Surg.* **2006**, *29*, 434–440. [CrossRef] [PubMed]
15. Jiang, X.; Xu, J.; Zhen, S.; Zhu, Y. Obesity is associated with postoperative outcomes in patients undergoing cardiac surgery: A cohort study. *BMC Anesthesiol.* **2023**, *23*, 3. [CrossRef]
16. Kitahara, H.; Patel, B.; McCrorey, M.; Nisivaco, S.; Balkhy, H.H. Morbid Oesity Dors not Increase Morbidity or Mortality in Robotic Cardiac Surgery. *Innovations* **2017**, *12*, 434–439. [CrossRef]
17. Mariscalco, G.; Wozniak, M.J.; Dawson, A.G.; Serraino, G.F.; Porter, R.; Nath, M.; Klersy, C.; Kumar, T.; Murphy, G.J. Body Mass Index and Mortality among Adults Undergoing Cardiac Surgery: A Nationwide Study with a Systematic Review and Meta-Analysis. *Circulation* **2017**, *135*, 850–863. [CrossRef]
18. Hartrumpf, M.; Kuehnel, R.-U.; Albes, J.M. The obesity paradox is still there: A risk analysis of over 15 000 cardiosurgical patients based on body mass index. *Interact. Cardiovasc. Thorac. Surg.* **2017**, *25*, 18–24. [CrossRef]
19. Kalantar-Zadeh, K.; Horwich, T.B.; Oreopoulos, A.; Kovesdy, C.P.; Younessi, H.; Anker, S.D.; Morley, J.E. Risk factor paradox in wasting diseases. *Curr. Opin. Clin. Nutr. Metab. Care* **2007**, *10*, 433–442. [CrossRef]
20. Carnethon, M.R.; Khan, S.S. An Apparent Obesity Paradox in Cardiac Surgery. *Circulation* **2017**, *135*, 864–866. [CrossRef]
21. Yasar, E.; Duman, Z.M.; Bayram, M.; Gürsoy, M.; Kadiroğulları, E.; Aydın, Ü. Obesity Does Not Affect Major Outcomes in Robotic Coronary Surgery. *HSF* **2023**, *26*, E525–E530. [CrossRef]
22. Reser, D.; Sundermann, S.; Grunenfelder, J.; Scherman, J.; Seifert, B.; Falk, V.; Jacobs, S. Obesity Should Not Deter a Surgeon from Selecting a Minimally Invasive Approach for Mitral Valve Surgery. *Innovations* **2013**, *8*, 225–229.
23. Pierpont, Y.N.; Dinh, T.P.; Salas, R.E.; Johnson, E.L.; Wright, T.G.; Robson, M.C.; Payne, W.G. Obesity and Surgical Wound Healing: A Current Review. *ISRN Obes.* **2014**, *2014*, 638936. [CrossRef] [PubMed]

24. Wang, T.J.; Parise, H.; Levy, D.; D'Agostino, R.B.; Wolf, P.A.; Vasan, R.S.; Benjamin, E.J. Obesity and the Risk of New-Onset Atrial Fibrillation. *JAMA* **2004**, *292*, 2471–2477. [CrossRef] [PubMed]
25. Xie, X.B.; Dai, X.F.; Qiu, Z.H.; Jiang, D.B.; Wu, Q.S.; Dong, Y.; Chen, L.W. Do obese patients benefit from isolated aortic valve replacement through a partial upper sternotomy? *J. Cardiothorac. Surg.* **2022**, *17*, 179. [CrossRef]
26. Deng, X.; Qin, P.; Lin, Y.; Tao, H.; Liu, F.; Lin, X.; Wang, B.; Bi, Y. The relationship between body mass index and postoperative delirium. *Brain Behav.* **2022**, *12*, e2534. [CrossRef]
27. Braun, C.; Schroeter, F.; Laux, M.L.; Kuehnel, R.U.; Ostovar, R.; Hartrumpf, M.; Necaev, A.-M.; Sido, V.; Albes, J.M. The Impact of Gender and Age in Obese Patients on Sternal Instability and Deep-Sternal-Wound-Healing Disorders after Median Sternotomy. *J. Clin. Med.* **2023**, *12*, 4271. [CrossRef]
28. Santana, O.; Reyna, J.; Grana, R.; Buendia, M.; Lamas, G.A.; Lamelas, J. Outcomes of Minimally Invasive Valve Surgery Versus Standard Sternotomy in Obese Patients Undergoing Isolated Valve Surgery. *Ann. Thorac. Surg.* **2011**, *91*, 406–410. [CrossRef]
29. Hadaya, J.; Sanaiha, Y.; Hernandez, R.; Tran, Z.; Shemin, R.J.; Benharash, P. Impact of hospital volume on resource use after elective cardiac surgery: A contemporary analysis. *Surgery* **2021**, *170*, 682–688. [CrossRef]

Disclaimer/Publisher's Note: The statements, opinions and data contained in all publications are solely those of the individual author(s) and contributor(s) and not of MDPI and/or the editor(s). MDPI and/or the editor(s) disclaim responsibility for any injury to people or property resulting from any ideas, methods, instructions or products referred to in the content.

Article

Hypothermic Ventricular Fibrillation in Redo Minimally Invasive Mitral Valve Surgery: A Promising Solution for a Surgical Challenge

Jawad Salman †, Maximilian Franz †, Khalil Aburahma, Nunzio Davide de Manna, Saleh Tavil, Sadeq Ali-Hasan-Al-Saegh *, Fabio Ius, Dietmar Boethig, Alina Zubarevich, Bastian Schmack, Tim Kaufeld, Aron-Frederik Popov, Arjang Ruhparwar and Alexander Weymann

Department of Cardiothoracic, Transplantation and Vascular Surgery, Hannover Medical School, 30625 Hannover, Germany; salman.jawad@mh-hannover.de (J.S.); schmack.bastian@mh-hannover.de (B.S.); weymann.alexander@mh-hannover.de (A.W.)
* Correspondence: al-saegh.sadeq@mh-hannover.de; Tel.: +49-176-1532-4895
† These authors contributed equally to this work.

Abstract: Background: Minimally invasive mitral valve surgery (MIMVS) is a treatment for severe mitral valve pathologies. In redo cases, especially after coronary artery bypass grafting (CABG) surgery with patent mammary bypass grafts, establishing aortic clamping followed by antegrade cardioplegia application might be challenging. Here, we present the outcome of hypothermic ventricular fibrillation as an alternative to conventional cardioprotection. **Methods**: Patients who underwent MIMVS either received hypothermic ventricular fibrillation (study group, $n = 48$) or antegrade cardioprotection (control group, $n = 840$) and were observed for 30 postoperative days. Data were retrospectively analyzed and collected from January 2011 until December 2022. **Results**: Patients in the study group had a higher preoperative prevalence of renal insufficiency ($p = 0.001$), extracardiac arteriopathy ($p = 0.001$), insulin-dependent diabetes mellitus ($p = 0.001$) and chronic lung disease ($p = 0.036$). Furthermore, they had a longer surgery time and a lower repair rate ($p < 0.001$). No difference, however, was seen in postoperative incidences of stroke ($p = 0.26$), myocardial infarction ($p = 1$) and mitral valve re-operation ($p = 1$) as well as 30-day mortality ($p = 0.1$) and postoperative mitral valve insufficiency or stenosis. **Conclusions**: The patients who underwent redo MIMVS with hypothermic ventricular fibrillation did not have worse outcomes or more serious adverse events compared to the patients who received routine conventional cardioprotection. Therefore, the use of hypothermic ventricular fibrillation appears to be a promising cardioprotective technique in this challenging patient population requiring redo MIMVS.

Keywords: redo minimally invasive mitral valve surgery; hypothermic ventricular fibrillation; outcomes

1. Introduction

Minimally invasive mitral valve surgery (MIMVS) has emerged as the treatment for severe mitral valve pathologies [1]. The development of MIMVS has been driven by advancements in surgical instrumentation, imaging modalities, and procedural approaches. Cardiac surgeons have refined and optimized techniques such as port-access, robot-assisted, and endoscopic-guided mitral valve interventions [1–3]. These minimally invasive methods have allowed for smaller incisions, reduced surgical trauma, and improved patient outcomes. Numerous studies have proven the feasibility and excellent outcomes of MIMVS when compared to traditional mitral valve surgery with full sternotomy [1–3].

Redo MIMVS represents a specialized and technically challenging surgical approach for patients requiring repeat interventions on the mitral valve. This technique is particularly beneficial for individuals who have previously undergone open-heart procedures, as it aims to mitigate the complexities and risks associated with repeat sternotomies [1,4–6]. In redo cases, especially after CABG surgery with patent mammary artery bypass grafts, it can be challenging to clamp the mammary bypass and establish aortic clamping followed by antegrade cardioprotection [2,7–9]. In situations where safely mobilizing the ascending aorta is not feasible, the use of an endoclamp can facilitate the surgical procedure. Alternatively, hypothermic ventricular fibrillation may serve as a viable option, as it allows the surgeon to operate on a protected heart while keeping the ascending aorta untouched [10,11].

In this study, we retrospectively analyzed the early postoperative outcomes of hypothermic ventricular fibrillation in redo minimally invasive mitral valve surgery.

2. Materials and Methods

2.1. Study Population and Design

Between January 2011 and December 2022, a total of 888 minimally invasive mitral valve surgeries were performed at our center. Among them, 48 patients received hypothermic ventricular fibrillation (study group), and 840 patients underwent antegrade cardioprotection (control group). Peri- and postoperative data were collected from our prospectively maintained database. Patient follow-up was conducted until the 30th postoperative day.

2.2. Ethical Statement

In accordance with local German protocols, study approval by the institutional ethical review board was waived given the retrospective and non-interventional design of this study.

2.3. Surgical Technique

The surgical technique has already been described elsewhere [12–14]. To sum up, single-lung ventilation was used, and cardiopulmonary bypass was usually established via the right inguinal vessels. First, a venous two-stage cannula was inserted over the right femoral vein into the superior vena cava under echocardiographic control. Then, the arterial cannula was inserted. All surgeries were performed via a right minithoracotomy. Carbon dioxide was insufflated during the whole procedure. The pericardium was opened 3–4 cm above the phrenic nerve. Hypothermia at 30 °C was induced by cardiopulmonary bypass which resulted in ventricular fibrillation. If this did not work, we also used electric shocks to induce fibrillation. Cerebral blood oxygen concentration was measured. Unfractionated heparin was intravenously applied to elevate the activated clotting time above 450 s, and after the removal of the venous cannula, antagonization with protamine was carried out. Postoperative transthoracic echocardiography was performed routinely before discharge and mitral valve function was evaluated. Stenosis was graded according to Omran et al. [15]. Insufficiency was graded as described by Chew et al. [16].

2.4. Outcomes Measures

The primary endpoint was 30-day mortality. Postoperative early mortality was defined as death occurring within the hospital stay and the first 30 days after operation. Secondary endpoints were the duration of postoperative intensive care unit (ICU) stay, as well as the incidence of postoperative ischemic stroke, right ventricular failure, new-onset atrial fibrillation, new-onset myocardial infarction, the need for pacemaker implantation, major bleeding requiring re-thoracotomy, sepsis, and renal failure requiring dialysis. Preoperative renal failure was attributed to patients who were diagnosed with acute or chronic renal failure by the referring hospital according to generally accepted parameters (decreased urine production, glomerular filtration rate).

2.5. Variables and Definitions

Variables were evaluated, including patient characteristics, further preoperative clinical assessments, laboratory parameters before surgery, intraoperative data, postoperative variables, and follow-up data. Elective, urgent, and emergency operations were performed, and the outcomes were compared between the groups. Elective patients were admitted routinely. Urgent patients were not admitted electively and needed to be operated on during the same hospital stay without the option to be sent home or already showed signs of heart failure. Emergency patients received surgery the same day the decision for surgery was made.

2.6. Echocardiographic Assessment

Preoperative and postoperative echocardiographic characteristics were analyzed, i.e., the preoperative left ventricular ejection fraction (LVEF), the rate of mitral valve insufficiency (MI) II, MI III and MI IV, as well as the rate of mitral valve stenosis (MS) II and MS III. The same characteristics were also analyzed postoperatively before hospital discharge.

2.7. Subgroup-Analysis

To explore the exact comparison, a sub-analysis was performed between the study group and the 7% of patients in the control group who had a history of cardiac surgery. The results are shown in the Supplementary Materials (Tables S1–S4).

2.8. Statistical Analysis

The data analysis was conducted using SPSS statistical software, version 28.01.1. For continuous variables, the results were summarized using medians and interquartile ranges. Categorical variables were described as the number of cases and the corresponding percentage relative to the overall study population. To compare continuous variables between groups, the Mann–Whitney U test was utilized. For categorical variables, Chi-square testing was employed. If any cell in the crosstab analysis had an expected count less than 5, Fisher's exact test was performed instead. A p-value less than 0.05 was considered statistically significant throughout the analyses.

3. Results

3.1. Baseline Characteristics

Patients from the study group had a median age of 70 years and patients from the control group had a median age of 67 years. Of all participants, 65% in the study group and 55% in the control group were male. All patients in the study group had undergone previous cardiac surgery (100%), compared to only 7% in the control group. The rate of preoperative CABG in the study group was 75%. One of the patients in the study group underwent transcatheter aortic valve replacement (TAVR), and another had a porcelain aorta, which is associated with a high risk of stroke during aortic clamping.

The distribution of pre-operative heart failure severity, as measured by New York Heart Association (NYHA) class, was similar between the two groups, with NYHA III being the most common in both groups. The timing of the procedures, whether elective, urgent, or emergency, was also comparable between the groups ($p = 0.09$). Patients in the study group had a higher prevalence of various comorbidities, including preoperative renal failure, extracardiac arteriopathy, chronic obstructive lung disease, insulin-dependent diabetes mellitus, pulmonary hypertension, coronary artery disease, arterial hypertension, hyperlipidemia, and atrial fibrillation.

Mitral valve regurgitation was the most frequent operative indication in both the study group (90%) and the control group (86%) ($p = 0.67$). However, the study group had a lower incidence of Carpentier type I (4% vs. 12%, $p < 0.001$) and Carpentier type II (21% vs. 56%, $p < 0.001$) mitral valve lesions. In contrast, they more often suffered from Carpentier type III lesions (42% vs. 17%; $p < 0.001$) (Table 1).

Table 1. Preoperative characteristics.

Variables	Study Group ($N = 48$)	Control Group ($N = 840$)	p-Value
Age	70 (65–76)	67 (56–75)	0.015
Male Gender	31 (65%)	459 (55%)	0.15
NYHA I	0 (0%)	36 (4%)	
NYHA II	14 (29%)	326 (39%)	0.42
NYHA III	27 (56%)	343 (41%)	
NYHA IV	2 (4%)	38 (5%)	
Elective operations	25 (52%)	547 (65%)	
Urgent operations	17 (35%)	237 (28%)	0.092
Emergency operations	6 (13%)	52 (6%)	
Cardiac re-operation	48 (100%)	60 (7%)	<0.001
Preoperative renal failure	22 (46%)	133 (16%)	<0.001
Extracardiac arteriopathy	13 (27%)	51 (6%)	<0.001
Chronic obstructive lung disease	13 (27%)	122 (15%)	0.036
Active endocarditis	2 (4%)	57 (7%)	0.75
Insulin dependent diabetes mellitus	11 (23%)	22 (3%)	<0.001
Recent myocardial infarction	1 (2%)	12 (1%)	0.52
Preoperative stroke	3 (6%)	69 (8%)	0.79
Preoperative neurologic symptoms	6 (13%)	88 (10%)	0.63
Pulmonary hypertension	32 (67%)	368 (44%)	0.003
Coronary artery disease	36 (75%)	217 (26%)	<0.001
Smoking history	12 (25%)	184 (22%)	0.60
Family history	3 (6%)	65 (8%)	1
Arterial hypertension	45 (94%)	555 (66%)	<0.001
Hyperlipidemia	40 (83%)	372 (44%)	<0.001
Atrial fibrillation	29 (60%)	376 (45%)	0.038
Mitral valve stenosis	3 (6%)	50 (6%)	0.76
Mitral valve regurgitation	43 (90%)	723 (86%)	0.67
Endocarditis	2 (4%)	41 (8%)	0.42
Mitral valve prolapse	14 (29%)	506 (60%)	<0.001
Mitral chord rupture	8 (17%)	363 (43%)	<0.001
Anulus dilatation	28 (38%)	418 (50%)	0.18
Carpentier I	2 (4%)	97 (12%)	<0.001
Carpentier II	10 (21%)	470 (56%)	<0.001
Carpentier III	20 (42%)	124 (17%)	<0.001

Continuous variables were described as the median and interquartile range. Categorical variables were described as mean with the related percentage.

3.2. Intraoperative Characteristics

The study group had a significantly longer overall surgical duration, with a median time of 235 min compared to 205 min in the control group ($p < 0.001$). However, the time spent on cardiopulmonary bypass was similar between the two groups, with a median of 154 min in the study group and 137 min in the control group ($p = 0.27$). The study group had a higher rate of biological valve replacement (54% vs. 24%, $p < 0.001$) and mechanical valve replacement (31% vs. 11%, $p < 0.001$) compared to the control group. Consequently, the mitral valve repair rate was lower in the study group (15% vs. 65%, $p < 0.001$), as were the rates of mitral valve plasty with neochordae (15% vs. 46%, $p < 0.001$) and cleft closure (0% vs. 9%, $p = 0.017$) (Table 2).

Table 2. Intraoperative data.

Variables	Study Group (N = 48)	Control Group (N = 840)	p-Value
Surgery time (min)	235 (200–265)	205 (176–240)	<0.001
Time on CPB (min)	154 (228–178)	137 (114–165)	0.27
Mitral valve replacement			
Biological	26 (54%)	201 (24%)	<0.001
Mechanical	15 (31%)	90 (11%)	<0.001
Mitral valve repair	7 (15%)	549 (65%)	<0.001
Plasty with neochordae	7 (15%)	390 (46%)	<0.001
Number of neochordae [§]	0 (0–0)	0 (0–2)	<0.001
Cleft closure	0 (0%)	82 (9%)	0.017
Segment resection	1 (2%)	40 (5%)	0.72
Sliding plasty	0 (0%)	5 (1%)	1
Augmentation	0 (0%)	33 (4%)	0.25
LAA closure	6 (13%)	246 (29%)	0.013
Maze procedure	3 (6%)	166 (20%)	0.021

CPB: cardiopulmonary bypass; LAA: left atrial appendage. Continuous variables were described as median and interquartile range. Categorical variables were described as number with the related percentage. [§] Data presented as medians and interquartile ranges.

3.3. Postoperative Characteristics

The time of postoperative catecholamine therapy (22 h vs. 17 h; $p < 0.001$), postoperative ventilation time (14 h vs. 11 h; $p < 0.001$), and time in the intensive care unit (4 days vs. 1 day; $p = 0.001$) were longer in the study group (Table 3). However, there were no significant differences between the groups in the rates of several postoperative outcomes, including the need for mitral valve re-operation (0% vs. 2%, $p = 1$); arrhythmias in general (21% vs. 11%, $p = 0.067$), including new-onset atrial fibrillation (10% vs. 10%, $p = 0.99$); pneumothorax (6% vs. 5%, $p = 0.74$); right ventricular failure requiring extracorporeal membrane oxygenation (ECMO) implantation (8% vs. 3%, $p = 0.084$); stroke (4% vs. 2%, $p = 0.26$); and cerebral bleeding (2% vs. 0%, $p = 0.26$). In contrast, the study group had a higher risk of postoperative complications, including a greater need for re-thoracotomy due to major bleeding (21% vs. 7%, $p = 0.07$) and pacemaker implantation (14% vs. 5%, $p = 0.016$). The study group also had a higher incidence of postoperative renal insufficiency requiring dialysis (13% vs. 3%, $p = 0.003$), although only 6% of the study group required ongoing dialysis after hospital discharge. The in-hospital mortality (6% vs. 2%, $p = 0.1$) and 30-day mortality (6% vs. 2%, $p = 0.1$) rates were similar between the two groups (Table 3). Out of the three deceased patients from the study group, one died due to sepsis, the second due to atherosclerotic mesenteric ischemia, and the third after suffering from postoperative low cardiac output syndrome. The first measured Creatine Kinase-MB (CK-MB) concentration was 61 (52–84) U/L in the study group and 51 (39–70) U/L in the control group. The lactate concentration was 1.6 (1.275–2.875) mmol/L in the study group and 1.4 (1–2) in the control group.

Table 3. Postoperative data.

Variables	Study Group (N = 48)	Control Group (N = 840)	p-Value
Catecholamine duration	22 (17–68)	17 (8–27)	<0.001
Ventilation time (h)	14 (10–33)	11 (7–16)	<0.001
ICU stay (days)	4 (1–6)	1 (1–3)	0.001
Mitral valve re-operation	0 (0%)	13 (2%)	1
Arrhythmia	10 (21%)	96 (11%)	0.067
Pneumothorax	3 (6%)	44 (5%)	0.74
ECMO/right ventricular failure	4 (8%)	27 (3%)	0.084
Re-thoracotomy due to Bleeding	10 (21%)	57 (7%)	0.01
New atrial fibrillation	5 (10%)	82 (10%)	0.99
Renal insufficiency with new onset dialysis	6 (13%)	23 (3%)	0.003
Stroke	2 (4%)	16 (2%)	0.26
Cerebral bleeding	1 (2%)	2 (0%)	0.15
Peripheral vascular complications	0 (0%)	5 (0%)	1
Sepsis	0 (0%)	12 (1%)	0.52
Myocardial infarction	0 (0%)	2 (0%)	1
Pacemaker implantation	7 (14%)	43 (5%)	0.016
30-day mortality	3 (6%)	18 (2%)	0.10
In-hospital mortality	3 (6%)	18 (2%)	0.10

ICU: intensive care unit; ECMO: extracorporeal membrane oxygenation. Continuous variables were described as median and interquartile range. Categorical variables were described as mean with the related percentage.

3.4. Echocardiographic Assessments

The preoperative echocardiographic assessment revealed that the study group had a lower left ventricular ejection fraction compared to the control group (56% vs. 60%, $p = 0.012$). However, the two groups were comparable in all other echocardiographic parameters evaluated, as shown in Table 4.

Table 4. Echocardiographic measurements.

Time	Variables	Study Group (N = 48)	Control Group (N = 840)	p-Value
Preoperative	LVEF	56 (44–62)	60 (53–65)	0.012
	MI II	11 (23%)	140 (17%)	0.92
	MI III	30 (63%)	563 (67%)	0.70
	MI IV	5 (10%)	78 (9%)	0.79
	MS II	1 (2%)	13 (2%)	0.53
	MS III	0 (0%)	23 (3%)	0.31
Postoperative	LVEF	55 (44–60)	53 (45–60)	0.74
	MI I	7 (15%)	155 (18%)	0.57
	MI II	0 (0%)	19 (2%)	0.62
	MI III	0 (0%)	1 (3%)	-
	MI IV	0 (0%)	0 (0%)	-
	MS II	0 (0%)	0 (0%)	-
	MS III	0 (0%)	0 (0%)	-

Continuous variables were described as median and interquartile range. Categorical variables were described as number with the related percentage.

4. Discussion

This retrospective study analyzed the early postoperative outcomes of redo MIMVS, where hypothermic ventricular fibrillation was used as cardioprotection. The study found that hypothermic ventricular fibrillation did not negatively impact 30-day mortality rates or the incidence of postoperative stroke and cerebral bleeding. However, our study did find a higher rate of postoperative renal failure requiring dialysis in the study group. It is important to note that these patients also had a higher prevalence of preexisting renal failure preoperatively. Furthermore, only half of the patients who required new onset dialysis postoperatively were under dialysis after hospital discharge. Additionally, the study group showed a higher rate of postoperative pacemaker implantation, which can be explained by the higher prevalence of preoperative atrial fibrillation in this group. Despite the high-risk profile of the patients in our study, the causes of death were primarily non-cardiac in nature.

Milani et al. analyzed ten patients who received MIMVS as reoperation with hypothermic ventricular fibrillation. Their results showed a 0% early postoperative mortality rate in this patient group [17]. According to our findings, the early postoperative mortality rate was 6%. However, two out of three deceased patients died due to mesenteric ischemia and sepsis, which were unrelated to cardioprotection. The third patient died due to postoperative low cardiac output syndrome. This patient was 75 years old and had preexisting NYHA Class IV heart failure. After the urgent mitral valve replacement procedure, the patient required veno-arterial (VA)-ECMO support for two postoperative days.

Romano et al. also investigated patients who underwent MIMVS with ventricular fibrillation as redo cardiac surgery. Their results showed a mean cardiopulmonary bypass time of 113 min, a mean postoperative ventilation time of 34 h, and a 30-day mortality rate of 7.4%. The stroke rate was 2.9%, and the incidences of sepsis, hemothorax, and renal failure requiring hemodialysis were 2.9%, 1.5%, and 1.5%, respectively [18]. In comparison with our findings, the current study's results showed a median cardiopulmonary bypass time of 154 min, a median postoperative ventilation time of 14 h, and a 30-day mortality rate of 6%. The stroke rate was 4%, and the incidences of sepsis, hemothorax, and renal failure requiring dialysis were 0%, 21%, and 13%, respectively. However, only 6% of patients were still on dialysis after hospital discharge. To sum up, 30-day mortality was comparable, although we had a higher rate of postoperative bleeding and requirement for postoperative new-onset dialysis.

A study by Davierwala et al. reported a 30-day mortality rate of only 0.8% after MIMVS. However, their cohort had a much lower rate of prior cardiac surgery at 5.4%. In contrast, the current study's patient population had a much higher rate of prior cardiac procedures, with 96% being cardiac redo cases [19]. Despite this, the 30-day mortality rate in our database was 6%, which is comparable to the 6.6% rate reported in the US STS database for mitral valve surgery after previous cardiac procedures [20]. Importantly, none of the deceased patients in the current study died due to the surgical procedure itself. The stroke rate of 4% in our study was also comparable to the 2% rate reported by Davierwala et al. [19]. However, the incidence of re-thoracotomy due to postoperative bleeding was higher in our study at 21%, compared to 7% in the Davierwala et al. study [19].

It should be noted that 75% of our patients who received MIMVS under ventricular fibrillation had undergone CABG with one of the bypasses being the left internal mammary artery to left anterior descending artery (LIMA-LAD), 17% had undergone previous valve replacement and one patient (4%) had previously received closure of an atrial septum defect. The difference in terms of previous cardiac procedures explains the seemingly higher complication rate of our study group. Additionally, a high incidence of preoperative renal failure (46% of our study group) naturally resulted in a higher demand for postoperative dialysis. Patients who underwent redo cardiac surgery were frequently under platelet inhibition or anticoagulation and, most importantly, had intrathoracic adhesions, all factors that tremendously increased the postoperative bleeding risk.

Hypothermic ventricular fibrillation in MIMVS provides a safe technique for high-risk patients who had already undergone cardiac surgery, such as CABG or valve replacement. In an aging population, it is a promising approach given the increasing number of patients who will undergo redo cardiac surgery. It also allows for a minimally invasive approach, preventing conversion to sternotomy, which is known to result in a longer postoperative hospital stay and is unpopular among patients [4].

One of the primary benefits of utilizing a right mini-thoracotomy approach for redo mitral valve surgery is the ability to avoid the risks associated with sternal re-entry and dissection of adhesions. This minimally invasive technique helps limit the potential for injury to cardiac structures or patent bypass grafts while also reducing the amount of postoperative bleeding [8]. Additionally, performing mitral valve surgery under ventricular fibrillation can help prevent the risk of systemic embolization that may occur with the use of aortic clamping, especially in patients with severe aortic calcification [21–23]. Current knowledge and our single-center experience suggest that MIMVS under hypothermic ventricular fibrillation without aortic cross-clamping through a right minithoracotomy is a safe, reproducible and effective option for patients requiring redo mitral valve surgery, especially when the patient has anatomical characteristics that increase the risk of re-sternotomy such as coronary bypass grafts.

5. Conclusions

The patients who underwent redo MIMVS with hypothermic ventricular fibrillation did not have worse outcomes or more serious adverse events compared to the patients who received routine conventional cardioprotection. Therefore, the use of hypothermic ventricular fibrillation appears to be a promising cardioprotective technique in this challenging patient population requiring redo MIMVS. The study has several limitations, including that the analysis was not performed using propensity score matching. In addition, the data only included the early follow-up period. To address these limitations, further studies with a larger patient cohort and long-term follow-up are required.

Supplementary Materials: The following supporting information can be downloaded at: https://www.mdpi.com/article/10.3390/jcm13144269/s1, Table S1: Preoperative characteristics; Table S2: Intraoperative data; Table S3: Post-operative data; Table S4: Echocardiographic measurements

Author Contributions: All authors contributed in the collection of data, manuscript development and Final approval. Conceptualization, J.S., A.W. and A.-F.P.; Methodology, M.F., K.A., T.K., N.D.d.M., S.T., F.I., D.B. and A.W.; Software, M.F., K.A., N.D.d.M., S.T., F.I., D.B. and A.Z.; Formal analysis, M.F., S.A.-H.-A.-S. and A.Z.; Validation, J.S., A.W., T.K., A.-F.P. and B.S.; Investigation, J.S., M.F., K.A., N.D.d.M., S.T., S.A.-H.-A.-S., F.I. and A.Z.; Writing—Original Draft Preparation, M.F., J.S., S.A.-H.-A.-S. and A.W.; Funding; T.K. and A.R.; Writing—Review and Editing, A.W., M.F., J.S., S.A.-H.-A.-S., A.Z. and B.S.; Supervision, J.S., A.R., A.W. and A.-F.P. All authors have read and agreed to the published version of the manuscript.

Funding: This research received no external funding.

Institutional Review Board Statement: In accordance with local German protocols, study approval by the institutional ethical review board was waived given the retrospective and non-interventional design of this study.

Informed Consent Statement: The study was conducted in accordance with the Declaration of Helsinki. Ethical approval was granted by the Medical School of Hannover's Institutional Review Board. Informed written consent was obtained from all participants, guaranteeing the confidentiality and anonymity of their data throughout the analysis.

Data Availability Statement: Data are contained within the article and Supplementary Materials.

Conflicts of Interest: Maximilian Franz received financial support from XVIVO which is unrelated to this work. Fabio Ius reports financial support from Biotest outside this study.

References

1. Akowuah, E.F.; Maier, R.H.; Hancock, H.C.; Kharatikoopaei, E.; Vale, L.; Fernandez-Garcia, C.; Ogundimu, E.; Wagnild, J.; Mathias, A.; Walmsley, Z.; et al. Minithoracotomy vs. Conventional Sternotomy for Mitral Valve Repair: A Randomized Clinical Trial. *JAMA* **2023**, *329*, 1957–1966. [CrossRef] [PubMed]
2. Güllü, A.; Şenay, Ş.; Ersin, E.; Demirhisar, Ö.; Whitham, T.; Koçyiğit, M.; Alhan, C. Robotic-assisted cardiac surgery without aortic cross-clamping: A safe alternative approach. *J. Card. Surg.* **2021**, *36*, 165–168. [CrossRef] [PubMed]

3. Kofler, M.; Van Praet, K.M.; Schambach, J.; Akansel, S.; Sündermann, S.; Schönrath, F.; Jacobs, S.; Falk, V.; Kempfert, J. Minimally invasive surgery versus sternotomy in native mitral valve endocarditis: A matched comparison. *Eur. J. Cardiothorac. Surg.* **2021**, *61*, 189–194. [CrossRef] [PubMed]
4. Eqbal, A.J.; Gupta, R.; Basha, A.; Qiu, Y.; Wu, N.; Rega, F.; Chu, F.V.; Belley-Cote, E.P.; Whitlock, R.P. Minimally invasive mitral valve surgery versus conventional sternotomy mitral valve surgery: A systematic review and meta-analysis of 119 studies. *J. Card. Surg.* **2022**, *37*, 1319–1327. [CrossRef]
5. Santana, O.; Larrauri-Reyes, M.; Zamora, C.; Mihos, C.G. Is a minimally invasive approach for mitral valve surgery more cost-effective than median sternotomy? *Interact. Cardiovasc. Thorac. Surg.* **2016**, *22*, 97–100. [CrossRef] [PubMed]
6. Kastengren, M.; Svenarud, P.; Källner, G.; Franco-Cereceda, A.; Liska, J.; Gran, I.; Dalén, M. Minimally invasive versus sternotomy mitral valve surgery when initiating a minimally invasive programme. *Eur. J. Cardiothorac. Surg.* **2020**, *58*, 1168–1174. [CrossRef] [PubMed]
7. Barbero, C.; Costamagna, A.; Verbrugghe, P.; Zacharias, J.; Van Praet, F.; Bove, T.; Agnino, A.; Kempfert, J.; Rinaldi, M. Clinical Impact of the Endo-aortic Clamp for Redo Mitral Valve Surgery. *J. Cardiovasc. Transl. Res.* **2024**. [CrossRef] [PubMed]
8. Botta, L.; Cannata, A.; Bruschi, G.; Fratto, P.; Taglieri, C.; Russo, C.F.; Martinelli, L. Minimally invasive approach for redo mitral valve surgery. *J. Thorac. Dis.* **2013**, *5* (Suppl. S6), S686–S693. [CrossRef] [PubMed]
9. Zwischenberger, B.A.; Gaca, J.G.; Milano, C.; Carr, K.; Glower, D.D. Late Survival After Redo Mitral Operation with Minithoracotomy Compared with Sternotomy. *Ann. Thorac. Surg.* **2024**, *117*, 353–359. [CrossRef] [PubMed]
10. Prestipino, F.; D'Ascoli, R.; Nagy, Á.; Paternoster, G.; Manzan, E.; Luzi, G. Mini-thoracotomy in redo mitral valve surgery: Safety and efficacy of a standardized procedure. *J. Thorac. Dis.* **2021**, *13*, 5363–5372. [CrossRef]
11. Murzi, M.; Miceli, A.; Di Stefano, G.; Cerillo, A.G.; Farneti, P.; Solinas, M.; Glauber, M. Minimally invasive right thoracotomy approach for mitral valve surgery in patients with previous sternotomy: A single institution experience with 173 patients. *J. Thorac. Cardiovasc. Surg.* **2014**, *148*, 2763–2768. [CrossRef] [PubMed]
12. Fleissner, F.; Salman, J.; Naqizadah, J.; Avsar, M.; Meier, J.; Warnecke, G.; Kuhn, C.; Cebotari, S.; Ziesing, S.; Haverich, A.; et al. Minimally Invasive Surgery in Mitral Valve Endocarditis. *Thorac. Cardiovasc. Surg.* **2019**, *67*, 637–643. [CrossRef] [PubMed]
13. Franz, M.; De Manna, N.D.; Schulz, S.; Ius, F.; Haverich, A.; Cebotari, S.; Tudorache, I.; Salman, J. Minimally Invasive Mitral Valve Surgery in the Elderly. *Thorac. Cardiovasc. Surg.* **2023**, *70*. [CrossRef] [PubMed]
14. Salman, J.; Fleissner, F.; Naqizadah, J.; Avsar, M.; Shrestha, M.; Warnecke, G.; Ismail, I.; Rumke, S.; Cebotari, S.; Haverich, A.; et al. Minimally Invasive Mitral Valve Surgery in Re-Do Cases-The New Standard Procedure? *Thorac. Cardiovasc. Surg.* **2018**, *66*, 545–551. [CrossRef]
15. Omran, A.S.; Arifi, A.A.; Mohamed, A.A. Echocardiography in mitral stenosis. *J. Saudi Heart Assoc.* **2011**, *23*, 51–58. [CrossRef] [PubMed]
16. Chew, P.G.; Bounford, K.; Plein, S.; Schlosshan, D.; Greenwood, J.P. Multimodality imaging for the quantitative assessment of mitral regurgitation. *Quant. Imaging Med. Surg.* **2018**, *8*, 342–359. [CrossRef] [PubMed]
17. Milani, R.; Brofman, P.R.; Oliveira, S.; Patrial Neto, L.; Rosa, M.; Lima, V.H.; Binder, L.F.; Sanches, A. Minimally invasive redo mitral valve surgery without aortic crossclamp. *Rev. Bras. Cir. Cardiovasc.* **2013**, *28*, 325–330. [CrossRef]
18. Romano, M.A.; Haft, J.W.; Pagani, F.D.; Bolling, S.F. Beating heart surgery via right thoracotomy for reoperative mitral valve surgery: A safe and effective operative alternative. *J. Thorac. Cardiovasc. Surg.* **2012**, *144*, 334–339. [CrossRef]
19. Davierwala, P.M.; Seeburger, J.; Pfannmueller, B.; Garbade, J.; Misfeld, M.; Borger, M.A.; Mohr, F.W. Minimally invasive mitral valve surgery: "The Leipzig experience". *Ann. Cardiothorac. Surg.* **2013**, *2*, 744–750. [CrossRef]
20. Kilic, A.; Acker, M.A.; Gleason, T.G.; Sultan, I.; Vemulapalli, S.; Thibault, D.; Ailawadi, G.; Badhwar, V.; Thourani, V.; Kilic, A. Clinical Outcomes of Mitral Valve Reoperations in the United States: An Analysis of The Society of Thoracic Surgeons National Database. *Ann. Thorac. Surg.* **2019**, *107*, 754–759. [CrossRef]
21. Crooke, G.A.; Schwartz, C.F.; Ribakove, G.H.; Ursomanno, P.; Gogoladze, G.; Culliford, A.T.; Galloway, A.C.; Grossi, E.A. Retrograde arterial perfusion, not incision location, significantly increases the risk of stroke in reoperative mitral valve procedures. *Ann. Thorac. Surg.* **2010**, *89*, 723–729; discussion 729–730. [CrossRef] [PubMed]
22. Svensson, L.G.; Blackstone, E.H.; Rajeswaran, J.; Sabik, J.F., 3rd; Lytle, B.W.; Gonzalez-Stawinski, G.; Varvitsiotis, P.; Banbury, M.K.; McCarthy, P.M.; Pettersson, G.B.; et al. Does the arterial cannulation site for circulatory arrest influence stroke risk? *Ann. Thorac. Surg.* **2004**, *78*, 1274–1284; discussion 1274–1284. [CrossRef] [PubMed]
23. Etz, C.D.; Plestis, K.A.; Kari, F.A.; Silovitz, D.; Bodian, C.A.; Spielvogel, D.; Griepp, R.B. Axillary cannulation significantly improves survival and neurologic outcome after atherosclerotic aneurysm repair of the aortic root and ascending aorta. *Ann. Thorac. Surg.* **2008**, *86*, 441–446; discussion 446–447. [CrossRef] [PubMed]

Disclaimer/Publisher's Note: The statements, opinions and data contained in all publications are solely those of the individual author(s) and contributor(s) and not of MDPI and/or the editor(s). MDPI and/or the editor(s) disclaim responsibility for any injury to people or property resulting from any ideas, methods, instructions or products referred to in the content.

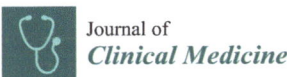

Journal of
Clinical Medicine

Article

Minimally Invasive Surgery through Right Mini-Thoracotomy for Mitral Valve Infective Endocarditis: Contraindicated or Safely Possible?

Maximilian Franz [†], Khalil Aburahma [†], Fabio Ius, Sadeq Ali-Hasan-Al-Saegh *, Dietmar Boethig, Nora Hertel, Alina Zubarevich, Tim Kaufeld, Arjang Ruhparwar, Alexander Weymann [‡] and Jawad Salman [‡]

Department of Cardiothoracic, Transplantation and Vascular Surgery, Hannover Medical School, 30625 Hannover, Germany; weymann.alexander@mh-hannover.de (A.W.); salman.jawad@mh-hannover.de (J.S.)
* Correspondence: al-saegh.sadeq@mh-hannover.de; Tel.: +49-176-1532-4895
[†] These authors contributed equally to this work.
[‡] These authors contributed equally to this work.

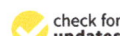

Citation: Franz, M.; Aburahma, K.; Ius, F.; Ali-Hasan-Al-Saegh, S.; Boethig, D.; Hertel, N.; Zubarevich, A.; Kaufeld, T.; Ruhparwar, A.; Weymann, A.; et al. Minimally Invasive Surgery through Right Mini-Thoracotomy for Mitral Valve Infective Endocarditis: Contraindicated or Safely Possible? *J. Clin. Med.* **2024**, *13*, 4182. https://doi.org/10.3390/jcm13144182

Academic Editors: Johannes Maximilian Albes and Manuel Wilbring

Received: 5 June 2024
Revised: 9 July 2024
Accepted: 15 July 2024
Published: 17 July 2024

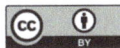

Copyright: © 2024 by the authors. Licensee MDPI, Basel, Switzerland. This article is an open access article distributed under the terms and conditions of the Creative Commons Attribution (CC BY) license (https://creativecommons.org/licenses/by/4.0/).

Abstract: Background: Mitral valve infective endocarditis (IE) still has a high mortality. Minimally invasive mitral valve surgery (MIMVS) is technically more challenging, especially in patients with endocarditis. Here, we compare the early postoperative outcome of patients with endocarditis and other indications for MIMVS. **Methods**: Two groups were formed, one consisting of patients who underwent surgery because of mitral valve endocarditis (IE group: $n = 75$) and the other group consisting of patients who had another indication for MIMVS (non-IE group: $n = 862$). Patients were observed for 30 postoperative days. Data were retrospectively reviewed and collected from January 2011 to September 2023. **Results**: Patients from the IE group were younger (60 vs. 68 years; $p < 0.001$) and had a higher preoperative history of stroke (26% vs. 6%; $p < 0.001$) with neurological symptoms (26% vs. 9%; $p < 0.001$). No difference was seen in overall surgery time (211 vs. 206 min; $p = 0.71$), time on cardiopulmonary bypass (137 vs. 137 min; $p = 0.42$) and aortic clamping time (76 vs. 78 min; $p = 0.42$). Concerning postoperative data, the IE group had a higher requirement of erythrocyte transfusion (2 vs. 0; $p = 0.041$). But no difference was seen in the need for a mitral valve redo procedure, bleeding, postoperative stroke, cerebral bleeding, new-onset dialysis, overall intubation time, sepsis, pacemaker implantation, wound healing disorders and 30-day mortality. **Conclusions**: Minimally invasive mitral valve surgery in patients with mitral valve endocarditis is feasible and safe. Infective endocarditis should not be considered as a contraindication for MIMVS.

Keywords: minimally invasive; mitral valve surgery; endocarditis; cardiac surgery

1. Introduction

Infective endocarditis can be considered a life-threatening infectious disease that affects the endocardium and heart valves. IE has an incidence of 3 to 10 per 100,000 patients per year, with a significant increasing trend [1]. Failure to promptly diagnose and manage IE can lead to high rates of morbidity and mortality. Complications associated with IE include heart failure, embolic events, abscess formation, sepsis, and septic shock [1–3].

The primary treatment for IE involves appropriate antibiotic therapy. When antibiotic therapy fails, mitral valve surgery plays a critical role in the management of infective endocarditis, particularly in cases with congestive heart failure, severe valvular regurgitation, persistent fever and bacteremia despite antibiotic therapy, systemic embolization, and large vegetations [1,4]. Over the years, significant advancements have been made in mitral valve surgery, with a growing emphasis on minimally invasive techniques with mini-thoracotomy approaches and progressing to robotic-assisted and video-assisted techniques [5,6].

In recent decades, the spectrum of indications for MIMVS has increasingly shifted and expanded to include more patients with a higher risk profile and more fragility and more complex mitral valve disease [4–6]. Careful patient selection is essential for the success of MIMVS [4–6]. Some surgeons consider endocarditis a contraindication for MIMVS based on several reasons, including, first, the limited access and reduced visibility associated with minimally invasive approaches, which may hinder the surgeon's ability to adequately visualize and debride infected tissue. Second is the complexity of endocarditis cases, including the presence of large vegetations, abscesses, or valve destruction, which may require more extensive surgical intervention best achieved through traditional sternotomy [4–6].

The purpose of this study is to report our long-term experience in the treatment of infective mitral valve endocarditis using MIMVS with right mini-thoracotomy.

2. Materials and Methods

2.1. Study Population

Between January 2011 and September 2023, a total of 892 minimally invasive mitral valve surgeries were performed at our center. Among these, 75 surgeries were conducted on patients diagnosed with active infective endocarditis of the mitral valve (IE group). The non-IE group consisted of 862 patients who underwent minimally invasive mitral valve surgery for other surgical indications. Peri- and postoperative data were collected from our prospectively maintained database. In accordance with local German protocols, study approval by the institutional ethical review board was waived given the retrospective and non-interventional design of this study.

2.2. Surgical Technique

The surgical technique used in this study has been previously described by Salman et al. [7]. In summary, single lung ventilation was used, and cardiopulmonary bypass was generally established through the right inguinal vessels. Initially, a venous two-stage cannula was inserted into the superior vena cava under echocardiographic guidance, followed by the insertion of an arterial cannula. All surgeries were performed via a right mini-thoracotomy, with continuous insufflation of carbon dioxide throughout the procedure. The pericardium was opened 3–4 cm above the phrenic nerve. Unfractionated heparin was administered intravenously to achieve an activated clotting time above 450 s, and protamine was used for antagonization after venous cannula removal. In cases where weaning from cardiopulmonary bypass (CPB) resulted in right ventricular failure, veno-arterial extracorporeal membrane oxygenation (ECMO) was established.

2.3. Follow-Up and Patient Data Collection

All patients were followed up for 30 days after surgery. Relevant clinical outcomes were recorded for all patients, including the incidence of postoperative ischemic stroke, right ventricular failure, new-onset atrial fibrillation, new-onset myocardial infarction, the need for pacemaker implantation, major bleeding requiring re-thoracotomy, sepsis, and renal failure requiring dialysis. Postoperative early mortality was defined as death occurring within hospital stay and the first 30 days after operation.

2.4. Echocardiographic Assessment

Baseline echocardiographic and hemodynamic evaluations were performed for all patients. Postoperative transthoracic echocardiography was routinely conducted prior to discharge to evaluate mitral valve function, with stenosis and insufficiency graded according to Omran et al. and Chew et al., respectively [8,9]. Pre- and postoperative echocardiographic features, including preoperative left ventricular ejection fraction (LVEF), rates of mitral valve insufficiency (MI) II, MI III, and MI IV, as well as rates of mitral valve stenosis (MS) II and MS III, were analyzed. The same features were also assessed postoperatively prior to hospital discharge.

2.5. Statistical Analysis

Data analysis was conducted using SPSS version 28.01.1. Continuous variables were described as the median and interquartile range (IQR). Categorical variables were presented as the number of cases and the percentage relative to the total group size. The Mann–Whitney U test was used to compare continuous variables, while the Chi-square test was employed for comparing categorical variables. Fisher's exact test was performed when at least one cell of the crosstab had an expected count less than 5. A p-value of less than 0.05 was considered statistically significant.

3. Results

3.1. Patient Characteristics

Patients in the IE group were younger compared to those in the non-IE group. They had a higher incidence of preoperative stroke and more frequent occurrence of neurological symptoms. In contrast, the IE group had a lower rate of preoperative pulmonary hypertension, coronary artery disease, arterial hypertension, hyperlipidemia, and atrial fibrillation. Mitral valve stenosis (0% vs. 7%; $p = 0.011$), severe mitral valve regurgitation (5% vs. 94%; $p < 0.001$) and annulus dilatation (23% vs. 50%; $p = 0.001$) were more prevalent in comparison with the non-IE group (Table 1).

Table 1. Preoperative data.

Variables	IE (n = 75)	non-IE (n = 862)	p-Value
• Preoperative characteristics			
Age	60 (50–69)	68 (58–75)	<0.001
Female gender	26 (34%)	400 (46%)	0.054
Cardiac reoperation	11 (15%)	96 (11%)	0.35
Chronic kidney disease	16 (21%)	148 (17%)	0.43
Hemodialysis	5 (7%)	35 (4%)	0.24
Extracardiac arteriopathy	2 (2.7%)	67 (8%)	0.16
Chronic obstructive lung disease	7 (9%)	133 (15%)	0.18
Recent pneumonia	0 (0%)	1 (0%)	1
Insulin dependent diabetes mellitus	2 (2.7%)	33 (4%)	0.84
Recent myocardial infarction	1 (1%)	12 (1%)	1
History of stroke	20 (27%)	54 (6%)	<0.001
Neurologic symptoms	20 (27%)	77 (9%)	<0.001
Pulmonary hypertension	14 (19%)	399 (46%)	<0.001
Coronary artery disease	11 (15%)	250 (29%)	0.01
Smoking history	13 (17%)	190 (22%)	0.38
Arterial hypertension	37 (49%)	591 (69%)	0.001
Hyperlipidemia	22 (29%)	401 (47%)	0.004
Atrial fibrillation	19 (25%)	405 (47%)	<0.001
• Operative indications			
Mitral valve stenosis	0 (0%)	57 (7%)	0.011
Mitral valve regurgitation	4 (5%)	809 (94%)	<0.001
Mitral valve prolapse	33 (44%)	513 (60%)	0.01
Mitral chord rupture	26 (35%)	355 (41%)	0.27
Anulus dilatation	17 (23%)	435 (50%)	0.001
Calcified anulus	0 (0%)	14 (2%)	1

3.2. Procedural Outcomes

There was no considerable difference in operation time, cardiopulmonary bypass time or aortic cross-clamp time between the groups. Patients in the IE group more often received mechanical valve replacement (24% vs. 10%; $p = 0.002$), while patients in the non-IE group more often underwent mitral valve repair (44% vs. 64%; $p = 0.001$) and concomitant tricuspid procedures (5% vs. 14%; $p = 0.033$) (Table 2).

Table 2. Intraoperative data.

Variables	IE ($n = 75$)	Non-IE ($n = 862$)	p-Value
Surgery time (minutes)	211 (172–251)	205 (176–239)	0.64
Time on CPB (minutes)	137 (114–180)	136 (113–164)	0.40
Aortic cross-clamp time	76 (61–104)	77 (59–95)	0.49
Mitral valve replacement			
Biological	24 (32%)	222 (26%)	0.27
Mechanical	18 (24%)	90 (10%)	0.002
Mitral valve repair	33 (44%)	550 (64%)	0.001
Concomitant tricuspid procedure	4 (5%)	122 (14%)	0.033

Postoperatively, there were no significant differences between the IE and non-IE groups in the incidence of stroke (3% vs. 2%; $p = 0.65$), intracerebral bleeding (1% vs. 0%; $p = 0.29$), delirium (4% vs. 3%; $p = 0.72$), sepsis (1% vs. 2%; $p = 1$), or new-onset myocardial infarction (0% vs. 0%; $p = 1$). The groups also did not differ in the rates of renal insufficiency with new-onset dialysis (5% vs. 3%; $p = 0.29$), right ventricular failure requiring ECMO (3% vs. 3%; $p = 1$), re-thoracotomy for bleeding (12% vs. 7%; $p = 0.11$), in-hospital mortality (4% vs. 2%; $p = 0.084$) or 30-day mortality (5% vs. 2%; $p = 0.24$). However, patients in the non-IE group had a higher postoperative incidence of new-onset atrial fibrillation (4% vs. 10%; $p = 0.002$) and arrhythmia in general (3% vs. 13%; $p = 0.005$), although there was no difference in pacemaker implantation rate (1% vs. 6%; $p = 0.12$) between the two groups (Table 3).

Table 3. Postoperative data.

Variables	IE ($n = 75$)	Non-IE ($n = 862$)	p-Value
Catecholamine duration	17 (6–39)	17 (9–27)	0.98
Ventilation time (hours)	11 (8–20)	11 (7–16)	0.12
ICU stay (days)	1 (0–2)	1 (0–2)	0.91
Mitral valve reoperation	3 (4%)	10 (1%)	0.81
Arrhythmia	2 (3%)	110 (13%)	0.005
Pneumothorax	2 (3%)	46 (5%)	0.42
ECMO/right ventricular failure	2 (3%)	29 (3%)	1
Re-thoracotomy/bleeding	9 (12%)	60 (7%)	0.11
New atrial fibrillation	3 (4%)	87 (10%)	0.002
Wound healing disorder	4 (5%)	57 (7%)	0.81
Renal insufficiency with new-onset dialysis	4 (5%)	26 (30%)	0.29
Stroke	2 (3%)	16 (2%)	0.65
Delirium	3 (4%)	26 (3%)	0.72
Cerebral bleeding	1 (1%)	3 (0.3%)	0.29
Periph. vascular complications	1 (1%)	4 (0.4%)	0.35

Table 3. *Cont.*

Variables	IE (*n* = 75)	Non-IE (*n* = 862)	*p*-Value
Sepsis	1 (1%)	14 (2%)	1
Myocardial infarction	0 (0%)	2 (0.2%)	1
Pacemaker implantation	1 (1%)	52 (6%)	0.12
30-day mortality	4 (5%)	18 (2%)	0.24
Intrahospital mortality	3 (4%)	17 (2%)	0.084

3.3. Echocardiographic Results

Postoperatively, there were no differences between the groups in ejection fraction (55% vs. 53%; $p = 0.74$), mitral valve insufficiency grade 1 (9% vs. 19%; $p = 0.1$), mitral valve insufficiency grade 2 (1% vs. 2%; $p = 1$), or mitral valve stenosis grade 2 (0% vs. 2%; $p = 1$). Mitral valve insufficiency grade 3 or 4, as well as mitral valve stenosis grade 3, were not observed in either group (Table 4).

Table 4. Echocardiographic measurements.

Time	Parameter	IE (*n* = 75)	Non-IE (*n* = 862)	*p*-Value
Preoperative	LVEF	60 (55–65)	60 (51–68)	0.012
	MI III	30 (40%)	568 (66%)	0.001
	MI IV	6 (8%)	77 (9%)	1
	MS II	0 (0%)	15 (2%)	0.62
	MS III	0 (0%)	26	0.03
Postoperative	LVEF	55 (45–60)	53 (45–60)	0.74
	MI I	7 (9%)	163 (19%)	0.1
	MI II	1 (1%)	20 (2%)	1
	MI III	0 (0%)	0 (0%)	-
	MI IV	0 (0%)	0 (0%)	-
	MS II	0 (0%)	20 (2%)	1
	MS III	0 (0%)	0 (0%)	-

4. Discussion

Over the past few years, there has been continuous development in the field of MIMVS. Experienced heart valve centers now routinely perform operations using a right mini-thoracotomy approach for complex valve diseases and high-risk patient subgroups, including those with infective endocarditis [5,10,11]. Despite the positive outcomes reported in the literature and the recognized advantages, the adoption of minimally invasive surgery for IE remains limited. Concerns have been raised regarding the challenges associated with the surgical learning curve, which could potentially compromise the effectiveness of the procedure and the ability to achieve optimal valve repair, particularly in complex valve diseases [11–13].

Our single-center retrospective analysis showed that patients from the IE group had a higher preoperative incidence of stroke and neurological symptoms, and mechanical valve prothesis was more often used in comparison to the non-IE group. However, the higher proportion of neurological disorders preoperatively was not reflected in the postoperative outcomes where the stroke rate in IE group was not more significant than in the non-IE group. Furthermore, the incidence of other postoperative complications including sepsis, myocardial infarction, right ventricular failure and renal insufficiency with new-onset dialysis in the patients of the IE group was low like in the non-IE group.

In a recent study by Barbero et al., positive early and long-term outcomes were reported in higher-risk patients who underwent minimally invasive surgery for mitral valve infective endocarditis [11]. The authors highlighted the crucial role of comprehensive screening, including total body, vascular and echocardiographic assessments, in selecting the most suitable approach [11]. This screening process enables the extension of indications for minimally invasive surgery to include patients with more severe conditions, such as active endocarditis and sepsis [11].

Folkmann et al. performed a retrospective, single-center analysis with a follow-up period of one year which analyzed the outcome of 92 patients who underwent MIMVS for mitral valve endocarditis [14]. They reported a mitral valve repair rate of 24%, postoperative stroke rate of 4%, sepsis rate of 2%, ECMO rate of 1% and dialysis rate of 13%. The 30-day mortality was 9.8% [14]. These results are slightly different from our results. We report a mitral valve repair rate of 44%, 30-day mortality of 5% and stroke, sepsis, ECMO and dialysis rates of 3%, 1%, 3% and 5%, respectively. To sum up, the complication rates in our study and in the study of Folkmann et al. are remarkably low, which confirms the safety and effectivity of MIMVS for mitral valve endocarditis.

Kofler et al. reported a shorter overall operation time, less blood transfusion and shorter ventilation time and finally concluded that the minimally invasive approach is superior to sternotomy in selected patients [15]. Their overall surgery time was shorter compared to the overall surgery time in the patients of our study, while their ventilation time was comparable to the ventilation time of the patients in our study group. The 30-day mortality was also identical.

Van Praet et al. stated in a case report that MIMVS for endocarditis reduces the risk of wound infections and consequently the risk of redo procedures [16]. We can confirm this statement through our results which show a wound infection rate of 5%. Van Praet et al., furthermore, stated that mitral valve replacement is acceptable if the endocarditis does not involve the anulus [16]. This is also in agreement with our work which has a replacement rate of 56% with a low rate of recurrence.

According to our findings and experience, MIMVS can hold great promise as an effective and less invasive treatment option for IE. This approach offers several important benefits, including reduced surgical trauma and better recovery with improved outcomes. To sum up, there is a limited amount of literature describing the short- and long-term outcomes after MIMVS in mitral valve endocarditis; however, the common statement of the available literature is clear: infective endocarditis should not be considered a contraindication for MIMVS, and the outcomes are clinically acceptable. Our work underlines this important statement.

5. Conclusions

Minimally invasive mitral valve surgery through right mini-thoracotomy for infective mitral valve endocarditis had no negative impact on the early postoperative outcome. Therefore, endocarditis should not be seen as a contraindication for minimally invasive mitral valve surgery. This study has several limitations that should be considered when interpreting the results. Firstly, the analysis was not conducted using propensity score matching. Additionally, the data only represented the early follow-up period, which could influence the results. To address these limitations, further research is needed to comprehensively compare the mid-term and long-term clinical outcomes of MIMVS in patients with IE versus non-IE.

Author Contributions: Conceptualization: A.W., A.R. and J.S.; Data curation: D.B., M.F., F.I. and K.A.; Formal analysis: M.F., D.B. and A.Z.; Investigation: F.I., K.A., N.H., T.K. and J.S.; Methodology: N.H., T.K., A.W., J.S. and A.Z.; Supervision: A.R., A.W. and J.S.; Writing—original draft: M.F. and S.A.-H.-A.-S.; Writing—review and editing: A.W. and S.A.-H.-A.-S. All authors have read and agreed to the published version of the manuscript.

Funding: This research received no external funding.

Institutional Review Board Statement: In accordance with local German protocols, study approval by the institutional ethical review board was waived given the retrospective and non-interventional design of this study.

Informed Consent Statement: The study was conducted in accordance with the Declaration of Helsinki. Ethical approval was granted by the Medical School of Hannover's Institutional Review Board. Informed written consent was obtained from all participants, guaranteeing the confidentiality and anonymity of their data throughout the analysis.

Data Availability Statement: The original contributions presented in the study are included in the article, further inquiries can be directed to the corresponding author.

Conflicts of Interest: The authors declare no conflicts of interest.

References

1. Jussli-Melchers, J.; Friedrich, C.; Mandler, K.; Alosh, M.H.; Salem, M.A.; Schoettler, J.; Cremer, J.; Haneya, A. Risk Factor Analysis for 30-day Mortality after Surgery for Infective Endocarditis. *Thorac. Cardiovasc. Surg.* **2024**, *ahead of print*. [CrossRef]
2. Rajani, R.; Klein, J.L. Infective endocarditis: A contemporary update. *Clin. Med.* **2020**, *20*, 31–35. [CrossRef] [PubMed]
3. Cahill, T.J.; Baddour, L.M.; Habib, G.; Hoen, B.; Salaun, E.; Pettersson, G.B.; Schafers, H.J.; Prendergast, B.D. Challenges in Infective Endocarditis. *J. Am. Coll. Cardiol.* **2017**, *69*, 325–344. [CrossRef] [PubMed]
4. Awad, A.K.; Wilson, K.; Elnagar, M.A.; Elbadawy, M.A.; Fathy, M.H. To repair or to replace in mitral valve infective endocarditis? an updated meta-analysis. *J. Cardiothorac. Surg.* **2024**, *19*, 247. [CrossRef]
5. El-Andari, R.; Watkins, A.R.; Fialka, N.M.; Kang, J.J.H.; Bozso, S.J.; Hassanabad, A.F.; Vasanthan, V.; Adams, C.; Cook, R.; Moon, M.C.; et al. Minimally Invasive Approaches to Mitral Valve Surgery: Where Are We Now? A Narrative Review. *Can. J. Cardiol.* **2024**. [CrossRef] [PubMed]
6. Bonatti, J.; Crailsheim, I.; Grabenwöger, M.; Winkler, B. Minimally Invasive and Robotic Mitral Valve Surgery: Methods and Outcomes in a 20-Year Review. *Innovations* **2021**, *16*, 317–326. [CrossRef] [PubMed]
7. Salman, J.; Fleissner, F.; Naqizadah, J.; Avsar, M.; Shrestha, M.; Warnecke, G.; Ismail, I.; Rumke, S.; Cebotari, S.; Haverich, A.; et al. Minimally Invasive Mitral Valve Surgery in Re-Do Cases-The New Standard Procedure? *Thorac. Cardiovasc. Surg.* **2018**, *66*, 545–551. [CrossRef] [PubMed]
8. Omran, A.S.; Arifi, A.A.; Mohamed, A.A. Echocardiography in mitral stenosis. *J. Saudi Heart Assoc.* **2011**, *23*, 51–58. [CrossRef] [PubMed]
9. Chew, P.G.; Bounford, K.; Plein, S.; Schlosshan, D.; Greenwood, J.P. Multimodality imaging for the quantitative assessment of mitral regurgitation. *Quant. Imaging Med. Surg.* **2018**, *8*, 342–359. [CrossRef] [PubMed]
10. Pojar, M.; Karalko, M.; Dergel, M.; Vojacek, J. Minimally invasive or sternotomy approach in mitral valve surgery: A propensity-matched comparison. *J. Cardiothorac. Surg.* **2021**, *16*, 228. [CrossRef] [PubMed]
11. Barbero, C.; Pocar, M.; Brenna, D.; Parrella, B.; Baldarelli, S.; Aloi, V.; Costamagna, A.; Trompeo, A.C.; Vairo, A.; Alunni, G.; et al. Minimally Invasive Surgery: Standard of Care for Mitral Valve Endocarditis. *Medicina* **2023**, *59*, 1435. [CrossRef] [PubMed]
12. Lalani, T.; Cabell, C.H.; Benjamin, D.K.; Lasca, O.; Naber, C.; Fowler, V.G., Jr.; Corey, G.R.; Chu, V.H.; Fenely, M.; Pachirat, O.; et al. Analysis of the impact of early surgery on in-hospital mortality of native valve endocarditis: Use of propensity score and instrumental variable methods to adjust for treatment-selection bias. *Circulation* **2010**, *121*, 1005–1013. [CrossRef] [PubMed]
13. Shih, E.; Squiers, J.J.; DiMaio, J.M. Systematic Review of Minimally Invasive Surgery for Mitral Valve Infective Endocarditis. *Innovations* **2021**, *16*, 244–248. [CrossRef] [PubMed]
14. Folkmann, S.; Seeburger, J.; Garbade, J.; Schon, U.; Misfeld, M.; Mohr, F.W.; Pfannmueller, B. Minimally Invasive Mitral Valve Surgery for Mitral Valve Infective Endocarditis. *Thorac. Cardiovasc. Surg.* **2018**, *66*, 525–529. [CrossRef] [PubMed]
15. Kofler, M.; Van Praet, K.M.; Schambach, J.; Akansel, S.; Sundermann, S.; Schonrath, F.; Jacobs, S.; Falk, V.; Kempfert, J. Minimally invasive surgery versus sternotomy in native mitral valve endocarditis: A matched comparison. *Eur. J. Cardiothorac. Surg.* **2021**, *61*, 189–194. [CrossRef] [PubMed]
16. Van Praet, K.M.; Kofler, M.; Sundermann, S.H.; Montagner, M.; Heck, R.; Starck, C.; Stamm, C.; Jacobs, S.; Kempfert, J.; Falk, V. Minimally invasive approach for infective mitral valve endocarditis. *Ann. Cardiothorac. Surg.* **2019**, *8*, 702–704. [CrossRef] [PubMed]

Disclaimer/Publisher's Note: The statements, opinions and data contained in all publications are solely those of the individual author(s) and contributor(s) and not of MDPI and/or the editor(s). MDPI and/or the editor(s) disclaim responsibility for any injury to people or property resulting from any ideas, methods, instructions or products referred to in the content.

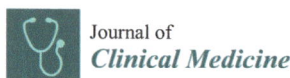 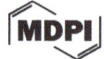

Review

Anesthesia for Minimal Invasive Cardiac Surgery: The Bonn Heart Center Protocol

Florian Piekarski [1,*], Marc Rohner [1], Nadejda Monsefi [2], Farhad Bakhtiary [2] and Markus Velten [1,3]

1. Department of Anesthesiology and Intensive Care Medicine, Rheinische Friedrich-Wilhelms-University, University Hospital Bonn, 53127 Bonn, Germany; marc.rohner@ukbonn.de (M.R.); markus.velten@utsouthwestern.edu (M.V.)
2. Department of Cardiac Surgery, Rheinische Friedrich-Wilhelms-University, University Hospital Bonn, 53127 Bonn, Germany; nadejda.monsefi@ukbonn.de (N.M.); farhad.bakhtiary@ukbonn.de (F.B.)
3. Department of Anesthesiology and Pain Management, Division of Cardiovascular and Thoracic Anesthesiology, University of Texas Southwestern Medical Center, Dallas, TX 75390, USA
* Correspondence: florian.piekarski@ukbonn.de

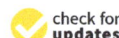

Citation: Piekarski, F.; Rohner, M.; Monsefi, N.; Bakhtiary, F.; Velten, M. Anesthesia for Minimal Invasive Cardiac Surgery: The Bonn Heart Center Protocol. *J. Clin. Med.* **2024**, *13*, 3939. https://doi.org/10.3390/jcm13133939

Academic Editor: Teruhiko Imamura

Received: 12 June 2024
Revised: 29 June 2024
Accepted: 3 July 2024
Published: 5 July 2024

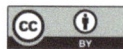

Copyright: © 2024 by the authors. Licensee MDPI, Basel, Switzerland. This article is an open access article distributed under the terms and conditions of the Creative Commons Attribution (CC BY) license (https://creativecommons.org/licenses/by/4.0/).

Abstract: The development and adoption of minimally invasive techniques has revolutionized various surgical disciplines and has also been introduced into cardiac surgery, offering patients less invasive options with reduced trauma and faster recovery time compared to traditional open-heart procedures with sternotomy. This article provides a comprehensive overview of the anesthesiologic management for minimally invasive cardiac surgery (MICS), focusing on preoperative assessment, intraoperative anesthesia techniques, and postoperative care protocols. Anesthesia induction and airway management strategies are tailored to each patient's needs, with meticulous attention to maintaining hemodynamic stability and ensuring adequate ventilation. Intraoperative monitoring, including transesophageal echocardiography (TEE), processed EEG monitoring, and near-infrared spectroscopy (NIRS), facilitates real-time assessment of cardiac and cerebral perfusion, as well as function, optimizing patient safety and improving outcomes. The peripheral cannulation techniques for cardiopulmonary bypass (CPB) initiation are described, highlighting the importance of cannula placement to minimize tissue as well as vessel trauma and optimize perfusion. This article also discusses specific MICS procedures, detailing anesthetic considerations and surgical techniques. The perioperative care of patients undergoing MICS requires a multidisciplinary approach including surgeons, perfusionists, and anesthesiologists adhering to standardized treatment protocols and pathways. By leveraging advanced monitoring techniques and tailored anesthetic protocols, clinicians can optimize patient outcomes and promote early extubation and enhanced recovery.

Keywords: anesthesia; minimally invasive cardiac surgery; management

1. Introduction

The development and implementation of minimally invasive techniques have significantly advanced various surgical specialties, including cardiac surgery. Minimal invasive cardiac surgery (MICS) offers patients less invasive approaches, resulting in reduced trauma and faster recovery time compared to traditional open-heart surgeries requiring sternotomy and its associated consequences, such as blood loss, infection, or increased postoperative pain [1–3]. MICS employs small incisions, specialized instruments, and advanced imaging technologies, enabling surgeons to perform intricate procedures with enhanced precision and minimal disruption to surrounding tissues. This reduces blood loss and, most notably, avoids sternotomies and their associated consequences [4].

The American Heart Association (AHA) defines MICS as surgical procedures performed through small chest wall incisions, typically thoracotomy, as opposed to traditional cardiac surgical procedures using sternotomy [5]. Consequently, catheter-based, transvascular approaches for structural heart diseases are not included in this scope. In addition to better cosmetic results [1], the advantages of MICS include reduced postoperative pain, a shorter hospital stay, and a lower risk of wound infection, bleeding, respiratory complications, and atrial fibrillation [2,3].

This approach has led to shorter duration of intensive care treatments, reduced hospital length of stay, and decreased incidence of hemodilution, bleeding, and the need for red blood cell (RBC) transfusion [6]. Furthermore, improvements in hematocrit, decreased post-operative pain, and a faster return to normal activities have been reported after MICS [7]. These findings mark a profound shift in perioperative cardiosurgical care. The number of MICS procedures continues to grow, encompassing a range of surgical techniques including bypass, valve, and aortic surgery, performed with the utilization or in the absence of cardiopulmonary bypass (CPB). A common feature of all MICS procedures is their performance in the absence of a sternotomy [4]. The expansive range of MICS includes minimally invasive direct coronary artery bypass (MIDCAB), valve repair and replacement, repair of septal defects, aortic procedures, and pulmonary vein ablation for atrial fibrillation [4,8].

The management of patients undergoing minimally invasive cardiac surgery requires not just detailed knowledge and experience regarding the corresponding procedure on the part of the surgeon, but also depends on a highly specialized cardio-anesthesiology team and established interdisciplinary treatment pathways.

At the Bonn Heart Center, a significant number of procedures are performed utilizing minimally invasive cardiac surgery (MICS) techniques. The presented recommendations are based on the current international literature and our institutional experience.

This article presents the anesthetic management for MICS on the basis of the Bonn Heart Center protocol and provides institutional treatment recommendations.

2. Preanesthetic Assessment

The objective of the pre-anesthesia assessment includes the assessment and evaluation of the patient's vascular access required for peripheral bypass cannulation. This varies depending on the corresponding procedure and anatomical variations, as well as relevant pre-existing conditions, including cardiac function, coronary artery disease, and pulmonary function [9]. An adequate risk stratification is carried out in order to optimize the patient's preoperative conditions. For planned surgeries, patients are evaluated by a cardiothoracic anesthetist at least one day prior to the procedure to identify potential contraindications and individual considerations. Some MICS procedures, such as minimally invasive direct coronary artery bypass (MIDCAB) surgery, require one-lung ventilation (OLV). Consequently, lung function tests and blood gas analysis are conducted, and the perioperative management is adapted accordingly.

It is essential to evaluate the presence of pulmonary hypertension and right ventricular dysfunction, as the utilization of OLV may potentially pose risks to these patients. Complications such as elevated pulmonary arterial pressure, heightened right ventricular afterload, and cardiac failure may arise as a result of OLV in this patient population [10].

Transesophageal echocardiography is of the highest importance for the echocardiographic guidance of minimally invasive cardiac procedures. Therefore, conditions of the upper gastrointestinal tract, in particular documented esophageal diseases, hiatal hernias, or previous operations and strictures, require evaluation. MICS is relatively contraindicated in cases of revision surgery, low cardiac output syndrome, or a severely reduced ejection fraction. The administration of sedative premedication is typically not included as part of the ERACS concept.

3. Induction

Following the implementation of standard hemodynamic monitoring, including electrocardiography (ECG) and pulse oximetry (SpO2), the left radial artery is cannulated under local anesthesia and ultrasound guidance. Subsequently, invasive blood pressure monitoring is conducted, and anesthesia is induced following preoxygenation with an opioid, such as remifentanil or sufentanil, a hypnotic agent (propofol), and a muscle relaxant (rocuronium). Anesthesia is maintained throughout the CPB procedure using volatile anesthetics, unless there is a suspicion of susceptibility to malignant hyperthermia or mitochondriopathy.

4. Airway Management

Following anesthesia induction and paralysis, endotracheal intubation is performed in accordance with a standardized institutional protocol, utilizing a single lumen tube for the majority of procedures. This is contingent upon a thorough assessment of the airway. The decision to employ video laryngoscopes is based on the results of the preoperative airway evaluation. The deflation of different lung parts is required, dependent on the performed MICS procedure. Various publications suggest lung isolation using a double-lumen endobronchial tube (DLT) or the utilization of a bronchus blocker. A prolonged duration of induction and total operative time has been observed in patients undergoing lung isolation by DLT, with no difference in the duration of ICU stay [11]. We utilize a single lumen tube for all on-pump MICS procedures and deflate both lungs after CPB has been established. Lung isolation using a left-sided DLT is established only for off-pump MIDCAB procedures. In this case, a left-sided DLT is the preferred option since right-sided DLTs have shown to be associated with poorer clinical performance [12]. Alternatively, in the event of a difficult airway, a single lumen tube is placed and then OLV is applied via bronchus blocker isolation of the lung. Lung deflation during MICS is associated with the potential occurrence of a pulmonary re-expansion edema, a rare but potentially catastrophic complication that may arise when the collapsed lung re-expands rapidly post-operation [13]. The sudden expansion can strain the pulmonary vasculature, leading to increased capillary permeability and fluid leakage into the interstitial spaces of the lung parenchyma. Consequently, patients may present with symptoms such as dyspnea, cough, and hypoxemia. It is important to understand the risk factors, including long CPB durations, diabetes, chronic obstructive pulmonary disease, right ventricular dysfunction, high pulmonary artery pressure, intraoperative fresh frozen plasma transfusion, and a high perioperative C-reactive protein level, and to implement preventive strategies during perioperative care [14]. These strategies play a pivotal role in mitigating the occurrence of pulmonary re-expansion edema, thereby optimizing patient outcomes following minimal invasive cardiac surgery. The use of total deflation has not resulted in an increase in the number of cases of clinically significant pulmonary edema that required invasive treatment.

5. Intraoperative Management

5.1. Monitoring

Irrespective of the surgical approach (minimally invasive or conventional), patients receive comprehensive cardio-anesthesiologic monitoring. Basic monitoring includes a five-channel ECG with ST segment analysis, SpO_2, $etCO_2$, temperature, invasive arterial blood pressure, central venous pressure, cerebral oximetry using near-infrared spectroscopy (NIRS), processed EEG (Bispectral Index (BIS)), and a comprehensive TEE evaluation. A pulmonary artery catheter is utilized in patients with pulmonary artery hypertension or right ventricular dysfunction. External defibrillation electrodes are applied, with the exception of off-pump coronary artery bypass (OPCAB) operations, as internal defibrillation with the internal shock paddles is difficult or impossible.

For central venous access, patients receive a 4-lumen central venous catheter, supplemented by a 9 FR venous catheter for volume access, typically inserted into the right internal jugular vein.

5.2. Transesophageal Echocardiography (TEE)

Comprehensive transesophageal echocardiography represents the gold standard for perioperative monitoring in cardiac surgery with some views being of central importance in minimally invasive cardiac surgery, given the potential contraindications [15]. Utilizing a comprehensive examination algorithm TEE facilitates assessment pre-, intra-, and postoperatively, enhancing surgical precision, confirming surgical indication, the positioning of bypass cannula, and patient safety.

5.3. Cerebral Oximetry

In the context of cardiac surgery, particularly in procedures with an elevated risk of cerebral ischemia, such as aortic surgery, which compromises the perfusion of the supra-aortic branches, near-infrared spectroscopy (NIRS) is a standard tool for the early detection of inadequate cerebral tissue oxygenation. It is essential to recognize that NIRS is associated with several inherent limitations. The optimal outcomes remain a topic of scientific investigation [16,17]. Cardiac surgery, particularly in procedures with heightened risks of cerebral ischemia, aortic surgeries affecting perfusion of supra-aortal branches, and near-infrared spectroscopy (NIRS) serve as vital tools for early detection of inadequate cerebral tissue oxygenation. Through continuous monitoring of cerebral oxygen saturation, surgical teams can promptly respond to potential complications, optimizing cerebral perfusion to mitigate the risk of neurological damage. Cerebral oximetry, an essential component of all cardiac procedures, ensures continuous, non-invasive assessment of cerebral blood flow dynamics. By discerning deviations indicative of compromised cerebral perfusion, cerebral oximetry informs management protocols outlined in a standardized approach. In particular, cerebral oximetry is advantageous in surgeries necessitating selective antegrade cerebral perfusion, such as aortic arch procedures, as it delivers indispensable insights into perfusion adequacy, enhancing surgical precision and patient safety.

5.4. Temperature Management

Temperature management is of paramount importance to coagulation and hemodynamic stability as well as in the context of ERACS [18]. The strategies employed are specifically adapted to align with the intended utilization of cardiopulmonary bypass (CPB) [19]. While the heart-lung machine can regulate patients' temperature during on-pump surgeries, significant temperature loss can occur during off-pump procedures. Therefore, passive as well as proactive warming measures, including prewarmed blankets, warming mats, and infusion warmers, are initiated prior to anesthesia induction for off-pump surgeries in the absence of CPB. Heat mats used alone or in addition to heat blankets have resulted in sustained body temperature even during prolonged off-pump bypass surgeries. Consequently, heat mats are employed for all off-pump procedures, whereas CPB is utilized to regulate body temperature during on-pump procedures and warming blankets are utilized pre- and post-bypass. Core temperature monitoring via bladder catheterization ensures precise temperature control throughout the procedure.

5.5. Peripheral Cannulation

The cannulation of peripheral vessels for the purpose of establishing cardiopulmonary bypass (CPB) in minimal invasive cardiac surgery requires a meticulous approach. This is necessary in order to facilitate optimal redirection of blood flow. The femoral artery and vein, as well as the right internal jugular vein, are commonly employed vessels for cannulation [9]. These vessels offer accessible peripheral entry points for the insertion of cannulas, allowing for the efficient initiation of CPB while minimizing trauma to surrounding tissues [20]. Furthermore, advancements in surgical techniques have enabled the utilization of peripheral vessels such as the axillary artery, providing alternative cannulation sites that further enhance the minimally invasive nature of the procedure. This is achieved by potentially beneficial antegrade flow during cardiac procedures, which is currently under investigation [21]. By carefully selecting and cannulating these vessels, surgeons can effectively establish CPB with precision and safety, thereby facilitating successful outcomes in minimal invasive cardiac surgery. For femoral veins, a lengthy cannula (Bio-Medicus 23/25 FR multistage femoral venous cannula, Medtronic, Minneapolis, MN, USA) is introduced into the inferior vena cava, primarily via the right femoral vein, with echocardiographic guidance (refer to Videos S1 and S2). According to the established protocol, the guidewires are visualized. The venous wire and cannula are depicted through TEE in the midesophageal bicaval view (see Figure 1a,b). The arterial wire is visualized in the descending aortic short-axis (SAX) and long-axis (LAX) views (see Figure 2 and Video S3). The exclusion of malposition such as in the hepatic vein or interatrial septum perforation is carried out.

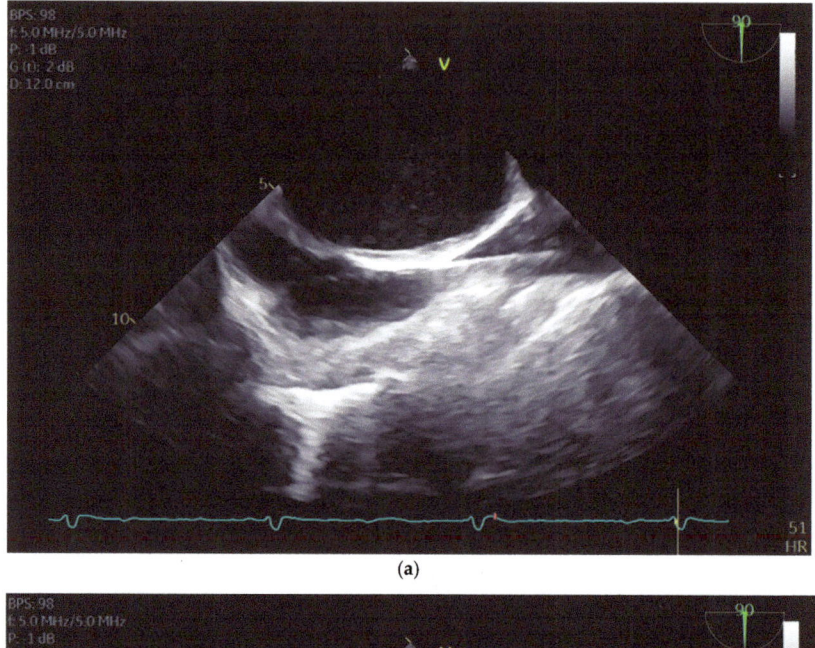

(a)

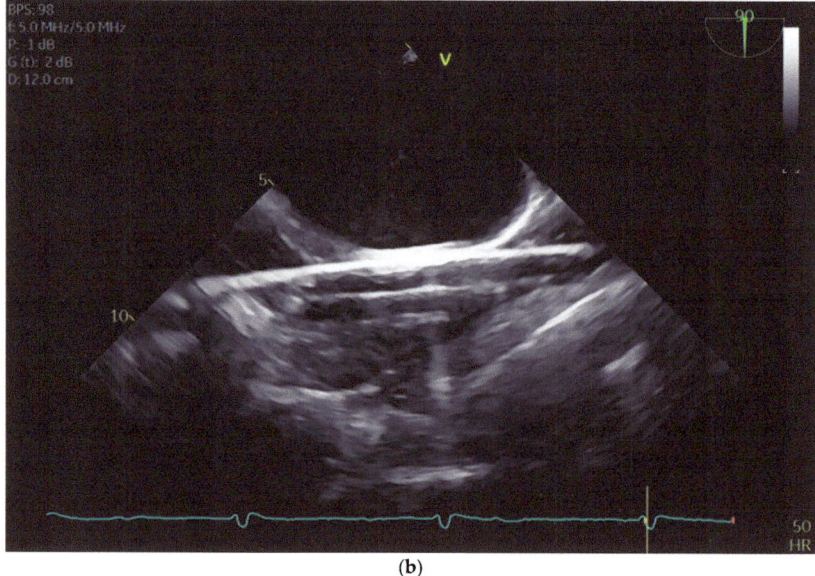

(b)

Figure 1. (a) shows the midesophageal bicaval view with the venous wire via the inferior vena cava into the superior vena cava; (b) shows the midesophageal bicaval view, with the cannula passing through the right atrium.

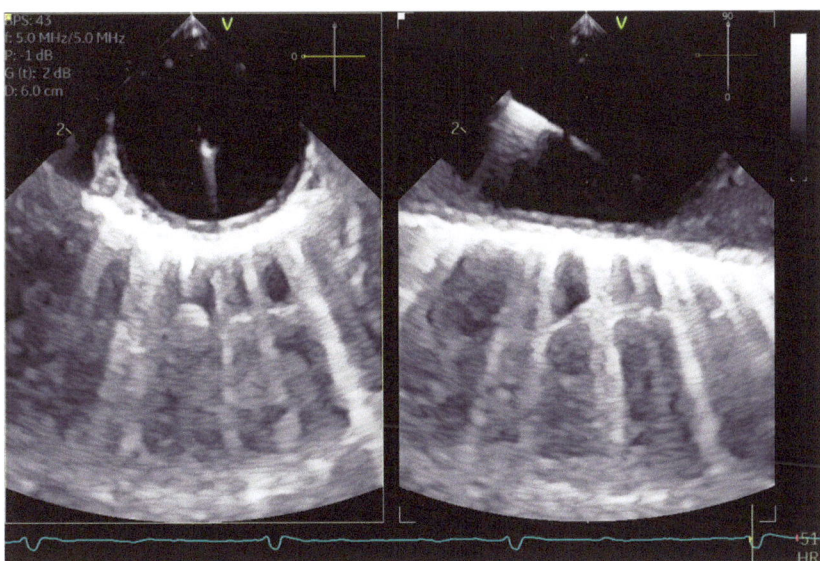

Figure 2. Shows the arterial wire in the descending aortic short-axis (SAX) and long-axis (LAX).

In certain cases, an additional cannulation of the superior vena cava (SVC) may be necessary, contingent on patient parameters such as body weight or specific surgical requirements, such as those pertaining to right atrial interventions. Indications for SVC cannulation include procedures requiring total bypass, such as tricuspid reconstruction/replacement, or procedures involving right atriotomy like ASD repair or mass resections for conditions such as tumors or thrombi. Furthermore, we perform SVC cannulation for all MICS procedures undergoing partial bypass in patients over 80 kg body weight for improved venous drainage.

The SVC drainage cannula (Edwards Fr 16/18 OptiSite arterial cannula) is placed via the right jugular vein under ultrasound guidance simultaneously with the central venous catheter insertion. The cannula is positioned caudally to the central venous catheter and other venous lines (see Figure 3a,b). It is important to note that cannulation is performed above the superior thorax aperture to avoid potential complications resulting from intrathoracic vascular damage. We do not perform side-separated cannulation of the central venous catheter and CPB cannula at our center. This approach offers advantages in terms of time management and protection of the contralateral side for possible subsequent punctures during hospitalization. No adverse effects were observed in association with the multiple access procedure.

The positioning of the wires and cannulas is meticulously executed exclusively under ultrasound guidance, in accordance with the center's policy and prevailing guidelines [22]. Prior to placement, the cannula is coated with 1 mL/2500 IU of heparin, with the objective of preventing immediate coagulation and clot formation subsequent to insertion. Following insertion into the internal jugular vein and after retrograde blood filling, the cannula is continuously flushed with a heparin-added full electrolyte solution (5000 IU heparin/500 mL) to sustain patency and prevent clot formation. A secure fixation is ensured with a pre-laid purse-string suture and a tourniquet is utilized to establish temporary fixation during the procedure. Post-completion of cardiopulmonary bypass (CPB) the remaining blood is flushed, the tourniquet is loosened, subsequently the cannula is carefully removed, and the incision site is closed using the pre-applied purse-string suture.

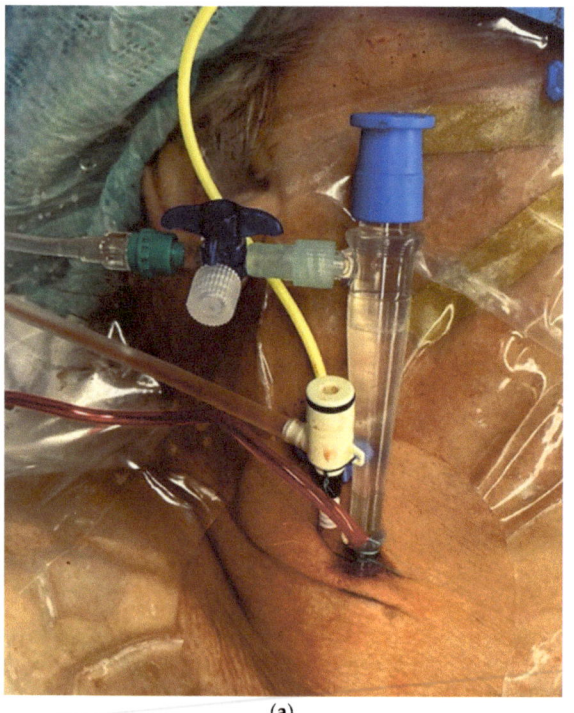

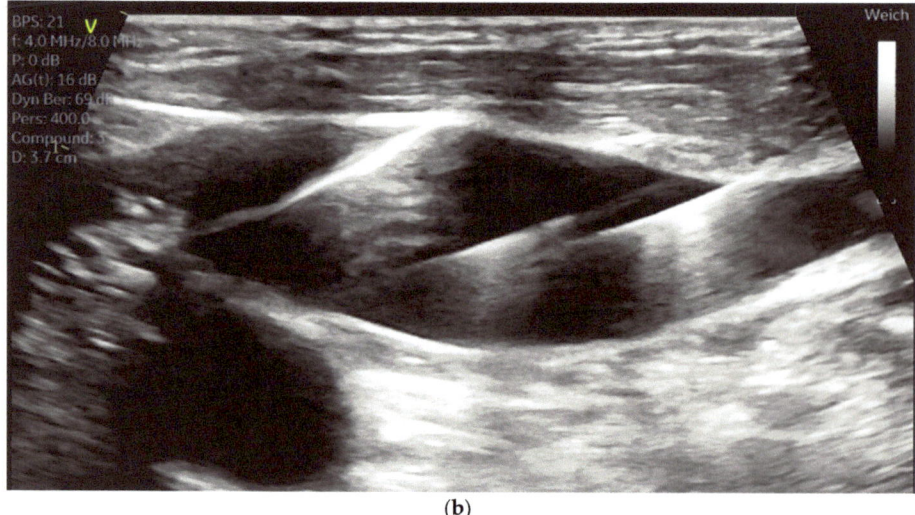

Figure 3. (**a**) shows the catheters inserted in the internal jugular vein right from cranial to caudal as follows: central 4-lumen central venous catheter, 1-lumen 9 FR catheter, and the CPB cannula; (**b**) shows three guidewires in the right internal jugular vein.

5.6. On-Table Extubation after Minimally Invasive Cardiac Surgery

Our anesthesiologic approach prioritizes on-table extubation (OTE) for MICS procedures in alignment with the Enhanced Recovery After Surgery (ERAS) concept [23–25]. Although randomized controlled trials on OTE are still pending, Jaquet et al. were able to demonstrate, in a retrospective analysis of 294 patients, that OTE was not associated with an increased incidence of respiratory complications and was associated with a lower risk of postoperative pneumonia and reduced requirement of vasopressors [19].

Preoperative screening allows for the identification of potential obstacles to on-table extubation. Subsequently, a comprehensive team evaluation precedes extubation. Extubation is initiated if the patient meets all criteria including adequate warmth, unobstructed gas exchange, competent coagulation, limited bleeding, and within-range vasopressor requirements. It is only performed if all team members agree at the end of the surgery. Weaning and extubation occur in the operating theater before patient transfer to the Intensive Care Unit (ICU).

5.7. MIDCAB

Minimally invasive direct coronary artery bypass graft (MIDCAB) surgery is a minimally invasive approach that is typically performed on the left anterior descending artery (LAD) at the front of the heart through a left-sided intercostal incision for left coronary artery access. However, this approach can also be utilized for the right coronary artery through a right-sided anterolateral minithoracotomy. Bypass grafting is performed on the beating heart and is typically employed for coronary grafts involving one or two vessels only. It is important to select the proper patients in order to achieve optimal results.

In order to ensure a direct and unrestricted view of the surgical field, OLV is employed for MIDCAB. This necessitates the use of a double-lumen tube for intubation, which enables lung isolation and selective ventilation. In accordance with our internal protocol, a bronchoscopy is conducted prior to skin incision to confirm the correct placement of the tube, with any necessary adjustments being made. As previously stated, a left-sided DTL is employed for all lung separations due to the reported inferior clinical performance of a right-sided DLT [12]. In cases where lung isolation is challenging, a bronchus blocker is utilized under bronchoscopic guidance as an alternative approach for lung isolation. While MIDCAB surgery is in general performed as an off-pump procedure at the beating heart it may occasionally be conducted utilizing mechanical support for patients with severely reduced ejection fraction. On this occasion peripheral cannulation is performed or a balloon pump is placed at the beginning of the surgery via femoral access. Temperature management is crucial and therefore warming is initiated prior to anesthesia induction using heating mats and blankets (Twinwarm BB and Universal III, MoeckWarmingSystems® Hamburg, Germany).

5.8. OPCAB

Off-pump coronary artery bypass (OPCAB) surgery is performed in the presence of sternotomy, and therefore does not formally count as part of minimally invasive cardiac surgery according to the AHA definition. However, we present the special features for anesthesia here, as these can be challenging.

In this technique, the surgeon performs coronary artery bypass grafting without stopping the heart or utilizing a heart-lung bypass machine. This approach offers potential benefits, such as a reduced risk of complications associated with cardiopulmonary bypass, reduced recovery times, and potentially better outcomes for certain patients compared to on-pump surgery. By avoiding the use of the heart-lung machine, OPCAB minimizes the systemic inflammatory response associated with conventional bypass surgery and reduces the risk of bleeding, potentially leading to faster postoperative recovery. OPCAB is often used to achieve the goal of reducing trauma to the patient and improving overall surgical outcomes. In some cases, for patients with severely reduced ejection fraction OPCAB can be performed under mechanical protection using cardiopulmonary bypass, IABP, or impella (on-pump beating technique).

Monitoring, anesthesia induction, and airway management are analogous to those of on-pump surgery. The anesthesiologist must address the hemodynamic fluctuations induced by heart positioning necessary for bypass grafting. This involves preload and afterload adjustments and administering vasopressors as warranted.

Off-pump CABG presents anesthesiologists with unique challenges that require precise management of hemodynamic stability through vasopressor application and targeted fluid management. Therefore, continuous cardiac function monitoring, hemodynamics, and end-organ perfusion are essential for early detection and prompt management of any deviations from the desired physiological parameters. Close interaction between all perioperative team members is imperative to ensure the successful outcome of off-pump CABG procedures. Maintaining adequate cerebral perfusion pressure is crucial for the prevention of POCD and delirium. The utilization of the Hypotension Prediction Index (HPI) parameter, developed by Edwards Lifesciences (Irvine, CA, USA), has been demonstrated to result in a reduction in critically low mean arterial pressure (MAP). The HPI is an algorithm based on the characteristics of the arterial pressure curve and has been shown to possess a high degree of sensitivity and specificity in predicting hypotensive episodes during cardiac surgeries [26].

5.9. Aortic Valve Repair/Replacement

The most common approach for performing aortic valve surgery is via a right anterior mini-thoracotomy. The surgical approach involves a limited skin incision and access through the third intercostal space, utilizing a soft tissue retractor for optimal exposure while preserving the integrity of surrounding structures such as the right internal thoracic artery and vein. Our institution utilizes an endoscopic approach. A 3D camera and Chitwood clamp are placed via the second intercostal space, with careful opening of the pericardium above the phrenic nerve to facilitate valve exposure [27]. This approach is safe and achieves excellent results in high-volume centers [28]. At our institution the standard protocol for this MICS procedure involves intubation and ventilation via a single lumen tube and total bilateral lung deflation after the establishment of CPB. This approach does not result in any restriction of the surgical field of vision [27], nor does it increase the risk of reperfusion edema compared to OLV.

Transesophageal echocardiography (TEE) is employed to evaluate the aortic valve preoperatively, with regard to the pathology. This includes determination of the valve opening area via the continuity equation and measurement of the aortic annulus for decision of prosthesis size. A three-dimensional annulus size assessment may be more adequate than two-dimensional. The guidance of the surgeon for peripheral puncture and cannula positioning is provided via TEE in the midesophageal bicaval view and the views of the descending aorta (SAX and LAX) [29].

Prior to termination of the cardiopulmonary bypass (CPB) procedure, the surgical result is verified by means of transesophageal echocardiography (TEE). Following completion of CPB, a re-evaluation is performed with a focus on valve function, the presence of new onset stenosis or regurgitation, as well as the occurrence of new ventricular movement disorders. The aorta is evaluated to exclude any dissection following de-clamping and de-canulation.

5.10. Mitral Valve Repair/Replacement

Endoscopic minimally invasive cardiac surgery (MICS) for mitral valve repair involves a 3–5 cm skin incision or peri-areolar approach above the right fourth intercostal space, aided by a 3D camera, to facilitate exposure of the mitral valve through incision via the interatrial groove and left atriotomy. Minimally invasive mitral valve procedures are conducted with great precision under the guidance of basic cardioanesthesia monitoring and meticulous vascular access protocols. For patients with a body weight exceeding 80 kg, a jugular cannula is carefully inserted into the right internal jugular vein and advanced to the innominate vein. The cannula insertion process is guided by echocardiography, ensuring accuracy and safety. Our center does not execute OLV during valve procedures.

TEE is used to perform a comprehensive evaluation of the mitral valve, pertaining to the pathogenesis of regurgitation in general and measuring the length of the anterior mitral leaflet (AML) and the mitral annulus for selection of the annuloplasty ring. Additionally, the potential for systolic anterior motion (SAM) is assessed via TEE.

Occlusion of the circumflex artery is a rare but serious complication after mitral valve surgery. The patency of the circumflex artery and regional wall motion abnormalities are evaluated by TEE [30].

5.11. Tricuspid Valve Repair/Replacement

Minimally invasive cardiac surgery for the tricuspid valve is performed concomitantly with mitral valve surgery. A total bypass is required for interventions on the tricuspid valve. Bicaval venous cannulation is performed through the external jugular and femoral veins, while arterial cannulation is performed through the common femoral artery. For the total bypass, bulldog vascular clamps are used for the superior and inferior vena cava. During the total bypass, vasoactive drugs are administered via the heart-lung machine.

5.12. Mass Resection

The advantages of MICS can also be utilized in the removal of benign or malignant cardiac masses. The choice of cannulation strategy depends on the location of the tumor. Intraoperative TEE plays a key role in determining and verifying the surgical results after removal of the tumor.

5.13. Bleeding

Minimally invasive procedures inherently involve small incisions, reducing the likelihood of extensive bleeding. The routine administration of coagulation factors is not recommended for these cases. However, in the event of bleeding not attributed to the surgical site, a prompt thromboelastographic assessment is conducted, followed by targeted optimization of blood coagulation.

Although the optimal dosing is still under investigation, tranexamic acid (TXA) is commonly used in cardiac surgery to reduce bleeding and the need for blood transfusions. At our institution tranexamic acid is administered as a standard protocol for all patients, with the exception of those undergoing MIDCAB surgery. A bolus dose of 10 mg/kg is initially administered, followed by a continuous infusion at 5 mg/kg/h. The anticoagulant effect of heparin is reversed with protamine, with real-time monitoring of activated clotting time (ACT) at the bedside to ensure optimal hemostasis.

5.14. Pain Management

At our center, we adopt a multifaceted approach to pain management. During surgery, either sufentanil or remifentanil is administered as opioids to effectively alleviate acute pain. The infiltration of the chest wall is carried out by the surgeon using a local anesthetic (10 mL 0.2% ropivacaine). Following surgery, peripheral analgesics (the first choice is metamizole (Novalgin®), or paracetamol as an alternative for metamizole allergy) are commonly employed to manage postoperative discomfort. Additionally, intravenous piritramide is available for pain relief as necessary. While regional anesthesia such as PECS II blockade is not routinely utilized, our comprehensive strategy is designed to minimize discomfort and facilitate early mobilization and recovery, ensuring optimal patient outcomes.

6. Conclusions

Minimal invasive cardiac surgeries have demonstrated excellent outcomes, with reduced morbidity, shorter recovery times, and improved patient satisfaction compared to traditional open-heart surgery at experienced centers. These results highlight the effectiveness and safety of MICS procedures in appropriately selected patients [31].

Anesthesia management is crucial for the outcome of minimal invasive cardiac surgery and requires careful consideration to ensure patient safety and optimal surgical conditions involving standardized treatment pathways. Overall, anesthesiologists must collaborate closely with the surgical team and perfusionists to address specific anesthesia implications related to cannulation strategies, hemodynamic management, lung isolation, temperature and fluid management, and coagulation control. Monitoring, including transesophageal echocardiography, is of great importance for the placement of catheters as well as for pre- and post-operative diagnostics. The management should be geared towards the earliest possible extubation with suitable patients.

Supplementary Materials: The following supporting information can be downloaded at: https://www.mdpi.com/article/10.3390/jcm13133939/s1, Video S1: ME bicaval guidewire passing RA; Video S2: ME bicaval cannula passing RA; Video S3: desc. Ao. Guidewire.

Author Contributions: Conceptualization, F.P. and M.V.; writing—original draft preparation, F.P. and M.V.; writing—review and editing; F.P., M.R., N.M., F.B. and M.V.; visualization, F.P., M.R. and M.V. All authors have read and agreed to the published version of the manuscript.

Funding: This research did not receive any specific grant from funding agencies in the public, commercial, or not-for-profit sectors.

Conflicts of Interest: FP has received support for professional training from Edwards Lifesciences and Abbott; MR has received support for professional training from Edwards Lifesciences and speakers' honoraria from Philips Healthcare; NM has no interests to be disclosed; FB discloses speakers' honoraria from Edwards Lifesciences, LSI, and Abbott; MV discloses speakers' honoraria from Edwards Lifesciences and Abbott.

References

1. Iyigun, T.; Kaya, M.; Gulbeyaz, S.O.; Fistikci, N.; Uyanik, G.; Yilmaz, B.; Onan, B.; Erkanli, K. Patient body image, self-esteem, and cosmetic results of minimally invasive robotic cardiac surgery. *Int. J. Surg.* **2017**, *39*, 88–94. [CrossRef] [PubMed]
2. Parnell, A.; Prince, M. Anaesthesia for minimally invasive cardiac surgery. *BJA Educ.* **2018**, *18*, 323–330. [CrossRef] [PubMed]
3. Aston, D.; Zeloof, D.; Falter, F. Anaesthesia for Minimally Invasive Cardiac Surgery. *J. Cardiovasc. Dev. Dis.* **2023**, *10*, 462. [CrossRef] [PubMed]
4. Ilcheva, L.; Risteski, P.; Tudorache, I.; Haussler, A.; Papadopoulos, N.; Odavic, D.; Rodriguez Cetina Biefer, H.; Dzemali, O. Beyond Conventional Operations: Embracing the Era of Contemporary Minimally Invasive Cardiac Surgery. *J. Clin. Med.* **2023**, *12*, 7210. [CrossRef] [PubMed]
5. Glauber, M.; Ferrarini, M.; Miceli, A. Minimally invasive aortic valve surgery: State of the art and future directions. *Ann. Cardiothorac. Surg.* **2015**, *4*, 26–32. [CrossRef] [PubMed]
6. Dieberg, G.; Smart, N.A.; King, N. Minimally invasive cardiac surgery: A systematic review and meta-analysis. *Int. J. Cardiol.* **2016**, *223*, 554–560. [CrossRef] [PubMed]
7. Baishya, J.; George, A.; Krishnamoorthy, J.; Muniraju, G.; Chakravarthy, M. Minimally invasive compared to conventional approach for coronary artery bypass grafting improves outcome. *Ann. Card Anaesth.* **2017**, *20*, 57–60. [CrossRef] [PubMed]
8. Goyal, A.; Chhabra, L.; Parekh, A.; Bhyan, P.; Khalid, N. Minimally Invasive Aortic Valve Surgery. In *StatPearls*; StatPearls Publishing: Treasure Island, FL, USA, 2024.
9. Lamelas, J.; Aberle, C.; Macias, A.E.; Alnajar, A. Cannulation Strategies for Minimally Invasive Cardiac Surgery. *Innovations* **2020**, *15*, 261–269. [CrossRef] [PubMed]
10. Ross, A.F.; Ueda, K. Pulmonary hypertension in thoracic surgical patients. *Curr. Opin. Anaesthesiol.* **2010**, *23*, 25–33. [CrossRef]
11. Kim, H.Y.; Baek, S.H.; Je, H.G.; Kim, T.K.; Kim, H.J.; Ahn, J.H.; Park, S.J. Comparison of the single-lumen endotracheal tube and double-lumen endobronchial tube used in minimally invasive cardiac surgery for the fast track protocol. *J. Thorac. Dis.* **2016**, *8*, 778–783. [CrossRef]
12. Kaplan, T.; Ekmekci, P.; Kazbek, B.K.; Ogan, N.; Alhan, A.; Kocer, B.; Han, S.; Tuzuner, F. Endobronchial intubation in thoracic surgery: Which side should be preferred? *Asian Cardiovasc. Thorac. Ann.* **2015**, *23*, 842–845. [CrossRef] [PubMed]
13. Irisawa, Y.; Hiraoka, A.; Totsugawa, T.; Chikazawa, G.; Nakajima, K.; Tamura, K.; Yoshitaka, H.; Sakaguchi, T. Re-expansion pulmonary oedema after minimally invasive cardiac surgery with right mini-thoracotomy. *Eur. J. Cardiothorac. Surg.* **2016**, *49*, 500–505. [CrossRef]
14. Moss, E.; Halkos, M.E.; Binongo, J.N.; Murphy, D.A. Prevention of Unilateral Pulmonary Edema Complicating Robotic Mitral Valve Operations. *Ann. Thorac. Surg.* **2017**, *103*, 98–104. [CrossRef] [PubMed]
15. Aybek, T.; Doss, M.; Abdel-Rahman, U.; Simon, A.; Miskovic, A.; Risteski, P.S.; Dogan, S.; Moritz, A. Echocardiographic assessment in minimally invasive mitral valve surgery. *Med. Sci. Monit.* **2005**, *11*, MT27-32. [PubMed]
16. Chiong, X.H.; Wong, Z.Z.; Lim, S.M.; Ng, T.Y.; Ng, K.T. The use of cerebral oximetry in cardiac surgery: A systematic review and meta-analysis of randomized controlled trials. *Ann. Card Anaesth.* **2022**, *25*, 384–398. [CrossRef] [PubMed]

17. Rogers, C.A.; Stoica, S.; Ellis, L.; Stokes, E.A.; Wordsworth, S.; Dabner, L.; Clayton, G.; Downes, R.; Nicholson, E.; Bennett, S.; et al. Randomized trial of near-infrared spectroscopy for personalized optimization of cerebral tissue oxygenation during cardiac surgery. *Br. J. Anaesth.* **2017**, *119*, 384–393. [CrossRef] [PubMed]
18. Maj, G.; Regesta, T.; Campanella, A.; Cavozza, C.; Parodi, G.; Audo, A. Optimal Management of Patients Treated With Minimally Invasive Cardiac Surgery in the Era of Enhanced Recovery After Surgery and Fast-Track Protocols: A Narrative Review. *J. Cardiothorac. Vasc. Anesth.* **2022**, *36*, 766–775. [CrossRef] [PubMed]
19. Jaquet, O.; Gos, L.; Amabili, P.; Donneau, A.F.; Mendes, M.A.; Bonhomme, V.; Tchana-Sato, V.; Hans, G.A. On-table Extubation After Minimally Invasive Cardiac Surgery: A Retrospective Observational Pilot Study. *J. Cardiothorac Vasc. Anesth.* **2023**, *37*, 2244–2251. [CrossRef] [PubMed]
20. Pozzoli, A.; Torre, T.; Toto, F.; Theologou, T.; Ferrari, E.; Demertzis, S. Percutaneous Venous Cannulation for Minimally Invasive Cardiac Surgery: The Safest and Effective Technique Described Step-by-Step. *Front. Surg.* **2022**, *9*, 828772. [CrossRef]
21. Kruse, J.; Silaschi, M.; Velten, M.; Wittmann, M.; Alaj, E.; Ahmad, A.E.; Zimmer, S.; Borger, M.A.; Bakhtiary, F. Femoral or Axillary Cannulation for Extracorporeal Circulation during Minimally Invasive Heart Valve Surgery (FAMI): Protocol for a Multi-Center Prospective Randomized Trial. *J. Clin. Med.* **2023**, *12*, 5344. [CrossRef]
22. Apfelbaum, J.L.; Rupp, S.M.; Tung, A.; Connis, R.T.; Domino, K.B.; Grant, M.D.; Mark, J.B. Practice Guidelines for Central Venous Access 2020: An Updated Report by the American Society of Anesthesiologists Task Force on Central Venous Access. *Anesthesiology* **2020**, *132*, 8–43. [CrossRef]
23. Salenger, R.; Morton-Bailey, V.; Grant, M.; Gregory, A.; Williams, J.B.; Engelman, D.T. Cardiac Enhanced Recovery After Surgery: A Guide to Team Building and Successful Implementation. *Semin. Thorac. Cardiovasc. Surg.* **2020**, *32*, 187–196. [CrossRef] [PubMed]
24. Ender, J.; Borger, M.A.; Scholz, M.; Funkat, A.K.; Anwar, N.; Sommer, M.; Mohr, F.W.; Fassl, J. Cardiac surgery fast-track treatment in a postanesthetic care unit: Six-month results of the Leipzig fast-track concept. *Anesthesiology* **2008**, *109*, 61–66. [CrossRef] [PubMed]
25. Zakhary, W.Z.A.; Turton, E.W.; Flo Forner, A.; von Aspern, K.; Borger, M.A.; Ender, J.K. A comparison of sufentanil vs. remifentanil in fast-track cardiac surgery patients. *Anaesthesia* **2019**, *74*, 602–608. [CrossRef] [PubMed]
26. Shin, B.; Maler, S.A.; Reddy, K.; Fleming, N.W. Use of the Hypotension Prediction Index During Cardiac Surgery. *J. Cardiothorac. Vasc. Anesth.* **2021**, *35*, 1769–1775. [CrossRef] [PubMed]
27. El-Sayed Ahmad, A.; Salamate, S.; Bakhtiary, F. Lessons learned from 10 years of experience with minimally invasive cardiac surgery. *Front. Cardiovasc. Med.* **2022**, *9*, 1053572. [CrossRef] [PubMed]
28. Bakhtiary, F.; El-Sayed Ahmad, A.; Amer, M.; Salamate, S.; Sirat, S.; Borger, M.A. Video-Assisted Minimally Invasive Aortic Valve Replacement Through Right Anterior Minithoracotomy for All Comers With Aortic Valve Disease. *Innovations* **2021**, *16*, 169–174. [CrossRef]
29. Kasel, A.M.; Cassese, S.; Bleiziffer, S.; Amaki, M.; Hahn, R.T.; Kastrati, A.; Sengupta, P.P. Standardized imaging for aortic annular sizing: Implications for transcatheter valve selection. *JACC Cardiovasc. Imaging* **2013**, *6*, 249–262. [CrossRef]
30. Ender, J.; Selbach, M.; Borger, M.A.; Krohmer, E.; Falk, V.; Kaisers, U.X.; Mohr, F.W.; Mukherjee, C. Echocardiographic identification of iatrogenic injury of the circumflex artery during minimally invasive mitral valve repair. *Ann. Thorac. Surg.* **2010**, *89*, 1866–1872. [CrossRef]
31. Monsefi, N.; Alaj, E.; Sirat, S.; Bakhtiary, F. Postoperative results of minimally invasive direct coronary artery bypass procedure in 234 patients. *Front. Cardiovasc. Med.* **2022**, *9*, 1051105. [CrossRef]

Disclaimer/Publisher's Note: The statements, opinions and data contained in all publications are solely those of the individual author(s) and contributor(s) and not of MDPI and/or the editor(s). MDPI and/or the editor(s) disclaim responsibility for any injury to people or property resulting from any ideas, methods, instructions or products referred to in the content.

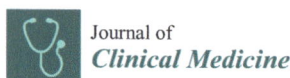 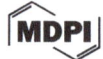

Article

Minimally Invasive Direct Coronary Artery Bypass Grafting: Sixteen Years of Single-Center Experience

Alexander Weymann [1,†], Lukman Amanov [1,†], Eleftherios Beltsios [1], Arian Arjomandi Rad [2], Marcin Szczechowicz [3], Ali Saad Merzah [1], Sadeq Ali-Hasan-Al-Saegh [1], Bastian Schmack [1], Issam Ismail [1], Aron-Frederik Popov [1], Arjang Ruhparwar [1] and Alina Zubarevich [1,*]

[1] Department of Cardiothoracic, Transplant and Vascular Surgery, Hannover Medical School, 30625 Hannover, Germany; merzah.ali@mh-hannover.de (A.S.M.)
[2] Medical Sciences Division, University of Oxford, Oxford OX1 2JD, UK
[3] Department of Cardiac Surgery, University Hospital Halle, 06120 Halle (Saale), Germany
* Correspondence: zubarevich.alina@mh-hannover.de; Tel.: +49-176-1532-4675
† These authors contributed equally to this work.

Abstract: **Background**: Coronary artery disease is a major cause of death globally. Minimally invasive direct coronary artery bypass (MIDCAB), using a small left anterior thoracotomy, aims to provide a less invasive alternative to traditional procedures, potentially improving patient outcomes with reduced recovery times. **Methods**: This retrospective, non-randomized study analyzed 310 patients who underwent MIDCAB between July 1999 and April 2022. Data were collected on demographics, clinical characteristics, operative and postoperative outcomes, and follow-up mortality and morbidity. Statistical analysis was conducted using IBM SPSS, with survival curves generated via the Kaplan–Meier method. **Results**: The cohort had a mean age of 63.3 ± 10.9 years, with 30.6% females. The majority of surgeries were elective (76.1%), with an average operating time of 129.7 ± 35.3 min. The median rate of intraoperative blood transfusions was 0.0 (CI 0.0–2.0) Units. The mean in-hospital stay was 8.7 ± 5.5 days, and the median ICU stay was just one day. Early postoperative complications were minimal, with a 0.64% in-hospital mortality rate. The 6-month and 1-year mortalities were 0.97%, with a 10-year survival rate of 94.3%. There were two cases of perioperative myocardial infarction and no instances of stroke or new onset dialysis. **Conclusions**: The MIDCAB approach demonstrates significant benefits in terms of patient recovery and long-term outcomes, offering a viable and effective alternative for patients suitable for less invasive procedures. Our results suggest that MIDCAB is a safe option with favorable survival rates, justifying its consideration in high-volume centers focused on minimally invasive techniques.

Keywords: MIDCAB; coronary revascularization; minimally invasive surgery

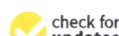

Citation: Weymann, A.; Amanov, L.; Beltsios, E.; Arjomandi Rad, A.; Szczechowicz, M.; Merzah, A.S.; Ali-Hasan-Al-Saegh, S.; Schmack, B.; Ismail, I.; Popov, A.-F.; et al. Minimally Invasive Direct Coronary Artery Bypass Grafting: Sixteen Years of Single-Center Experience. *J. Clin. Med.* **2024**, *13*, 3338. https://doi.org/10.3390/jcm13113338

Academic Editor: Manuel Wilbring

Received: 30 April 2024
Revised: 29 May 2024
Accepted: 3 June 2024
Published: 5 June 2024

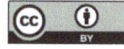

Copyright: © 2024 by the authors. Licensee MDPI, Basel, Switzerland. This article is an open access article distributed under the terms and conditions of the Creative Commons Attribution (CC BY) license (https://creativecommons.org/licenses/by/4.0/).

1. Introduction

Coronary artery disease stands as one of the leading causes of death in Western nations. The inception of coronary artery bypass grafting (CABG) in the 1960s marked its swift ascent to being amongst the most frequently conducted surgical interventions [1]. Over the years, significant improvements in outcomes have been observed, marked by reductions in both operative mortality and major morbidity rates [2]. Although outcomes have improved significantly in recent decades, the aging demographic of cardiac surgery patients, coupled with their increased comorbidities, has highlighted the necessity for less invasive surgical techniques [3]. Technological and engineering advancements over the last few decades have paved the way for the development of minimally invasive surgical methods, including the use of endoscopy in various procedures such as cardiac surgery [4]. Amongst the new perspectives in cardiac surgery, an alternative approach to a standard sternotomy for CABG has been implemented in recent years to facilitate a minimally invasive direct coronary artery bypass (MIDCAB) through a small left anterior thoracotomy. The left internal mammary artery (LIMA) can then be harvested either via direct vision or using endoscopic techniques [2]. Although the MIDCAB approach is commonly associated with increased postoperative pain for the patients, recovery appears to be faster than after a sternotomy, with potential improvement in the overall postoperative quality of life for the patients [2].

The MIDCAB approach may offer promising benefits for patients requiring surgical myocardial revascularization. However, its technically demanding nature and the lack of long-term outcomes remain major burdens for its further adoption [5]. The purpose of this retrospective study is to review and present the results of our single-center experience with MIDCAB for surgical myocardial revascularization.

2. Materials and Methods

2.1. Study Design

This study is a single-centered, retrospective, nonrandomized study including 310 patients who underwent a MIDCAB operation between July 1999 and April 2022 at our institution.

2.2. Inclusion Criteria—Population

Every patient who underwent a MIDCAB operation at our institution between July 1999 and April 2022 was eligible for this study. Both elective, urgent, and emergent cases were included in the present study. The decision to perform a MIDCAB operation was individualized for each patient based on the coronary anatomy and was made at the surgeons' discretion, always in accordance with the latest guidelines, our institutional multidisciplinary Heart Team decision, and patients' informed consent.

2.3. Operative Technique

Under general anesthesia and with single-lumen intubation, the patient was placed on the operating table in a supine position with a slightly elevated left scapula. A small (5–8 cm) anterolateral thoracotomy was performed in the left fourth intercostal space. Transesophageal echocardiography and ECG were used to monitor ventricular function throughout the procedure. A specialized rib retractor (Thoralift™ and, in the most recent cases, Mutistation™, LSI Solutions, Victor, NY, USA) was selected to partially elevate the rib cage to achieve better visibility during LIMA harvesting. In order to achieve a sufficient length to reach the coronary artery without tension, the artery was mobilized to the highest possible level (up to the subclavian vein). Heparin was administered intravenously until the target PTT of >300 s had been reached. A stabilization device (Octopus™, Medtronic, Minneapolis, MN, USA) was positioned to expose the LAD, and a longitudinal incision was made in the coronary artery. The LIMA graft was carefully prepared for the bypass. A shunt was placed into the coronary vessel and the end-to-side anastomosis was performed with 7/0 polypropylene (Prolene™) suture in a running fashion. The shunt was removed, and the anastomosis was completed. The bulldog clamp was removed from the LIMA and the coronary flow was restored. Heparin was reversed and after completing the flow measurement, the wound was closed in anatomic layers. The patient was delivered intubated to the intensive care unit to be extubated in the following hours.

2.4. Data Acquisition

In accordance with the data protection regulations, demographic information, clinical characteristics, and operative and postoperative data were retrospectively extracted from the institutional medical records of the included patients. Telephone interviews with the patients or/and their relatives or/and their primary care physicians were performed for an active follow-up.

Due to the retrospective, observation nature of the study, the requirement for informed consent was deferred. This study was performed in accordance with the Declaration of Helsinki, and the data regarding the patient's identity remained strictly anonymous. Ethical approval was obtained from the Ethics Committee of the Hannover Medical School,

Hannover, Germany (Nr.11333_BO_K_2024, 4 April 2024). All methods utilized in the present study were performed in accordance with regulations and guidelines.

2.5. Definitions and Outcomes

The primary endpoints of the present study were 30-day, 6-month, and 1-year mortality, as well as the overall survival at 5 and 10 years. The main secondary endpoint was the development of any postoperative adverse events. Data regarding the in-hospital stay, the intraoperative time, the need for transfusion, total ventilation time, conversion to sternotomy, and the need for surgical revision were also retrospectively retrieved. Urgent procedures were defined as procedures which had to be performed during the first 48 h after hospital admission. Emergent procedures were defined as procedures which had to be performed during the first 2 h after hospital admission.

Postoperative myocardial infarction was defined as a significant elevation of the CK-MB levels over 10% of the CK levels and a clinical correlate such as new changes in the ECG (ST-elevation or T-depression) and/or new dyskinesia detected by echocardiography. Hyperlipoproteinemia was defined as a state of abnormally high levels of triglycerides in blood (>150 mg/dL), requiring medical therapy. Kidney function impairment was defined as a reduction in GRF rate under 50 mL/min.

2.6. Statistical Analysis

The obtained data were entered into a dedicated Microsoft Excel spreadsheet. Statistical analysis was performed using IBM SPSS version 28 (IBM Corp., Chicago, IL, USA). Data were tested for normality using the Shapiro–Wilk test. When the data were not normally distributed, continuous variables were expressed as medians (interquartile range, IQR) or as mean ± standard deviation. Survival curves were generated using the Kaplan–Meier method. Categorical variables were expressed as frequencies and percentages.

3. Results

3.1. Baseline Characteristics

The mean age of the patients was 63.3 ± 10.9 years, and 30.6% of the patients were female (Table 1). All patients presented with symptomatic coronary artery disease, with 5.4% of the patients (n = 17) suffering from acute myocardial infarction. Interestingly, the EuroSCORE II rates in those seventeen patients did not significantly differ from the rest of the cohort; therefore, there was no hesitation in performing the procedure via minimally invasive access. A large portion of the cohort (73 patients (23.5%)) had previously undergone a PCI, 30% of the patients were active smokers, and 57 patients (18.4%) were suffering from type 2 diabetes mellitus. The patients presented with a mean left ventricular ejection fraction of 57.1 ± 6.5 and a median EuroSCORE II of 0.9 (0.7–1.2), putting the patients into the low-risk group. Further details of patients' baseline data are presented in Table 1.

Table 1. Baseline characteristics.

Parameter	n (%)
age	63.3 ± 10.9
female gender	95 (30.6%)
CAD1	197 (63.5%)
CAD2	71 (22.9%)
CAD3	42 (13.5%)
acute STEMI	2 (0.6%)
acute NSTEMI	15 (4.8%)
previous PCI	73 (23.5%)
active smoker	93 (30%)
IDDM	9 (2.9%)
NIDDM	48 (15.5%)
hyperlipoproteinemia	160 (51.6%)

Table 1. Cont.

Parameter	n (%)
arterial hypertension	280 (90.3%)
kidney function impairment	25 (8.1%)
terminal KI with dialysis	3 (1%)
LVEF, %	57.1 ± 6.5
EuroSCORE II, %	0.9 (0.7–1.2)

CAD—coronary artery disease, STEMI—ST-elevation myocardial infarction, NSTEMI—non-ST-elevation myocardial infarction, IDDM—insulin-dependent diabetes mellitus, KI—kidney injury, LVEF—left ventricular ejection fraction, and NIDDM—non-insulin-dependent diabetes mellitus.

3.2. Intraoperative Characteristics

In all cases, one anastomosis was performed (left internal mammary artery to ramus interventricularis anterior) on the beating heart without the cardiopulmonary bypass support. In 1% of the patients (n = 3), due to the problems with the anastomosis, the procedure had to be switched to a median sternotomy, and the anastomosis was performed on-pump with a beating heart. None of the patients had been considered for hybrid revascularization.

The mean operating time was 129.7 ± 35.3 min, and in most cases, the median rate of intraoperative blood transfusions was 0.0 (CI 0.0–2.0) Units with a mean requirement of 0.35 Units per patient. The majority of the cases were elective (76.1%). Further intraoperative data are presented in Table 2.

Table 2. Intraoperative data.

Parameter	n (%)
urgency	
elective	236 (76.1%)
urgency	61 (19.7%)
emergent	13 (4.2%)
MIDCAB (LIMA-LAD)	310 (100%)
operating time, min	129.7 ± 35.3
conversion to sternotomy	3 (1%)
conversion to CPB	3 (1%)
blood transfusion, Units	0.0 (0.0–2.0)
blood transfusion	87 (28.0%)

CPB—cardiopulmonary bypass, LAD—left anterior descending, LIMA—left internal mammary artery, and MIDCAB—minimally invasive direct coronary artery bypass.

3.3. Overall Survival and Postoperative Outcomes

The mean in-hospital stay duration was 8.7 ± 5.5 days and the median ICU-stay duration was 1(0.-1.0) day. Two patients suffered from perioperative myocardial infarction (0.67%), and in those cases, coronary angiography was performed. There were no cases of stroke in our cohort, and in four cases (1.3%), re-exploration for bleeding was necessary. There was no relevant need for postoperative blood transfusion in our cohort (Table 3).

Table 3. Postoperative data.

Parameter	n (%)
in-hospital stay, days	8.7 ± 5.5
ICU stay, days	1.0 (0–1.0)
new onset AF	7 (2.3%)
max CK	577.5 ± 430.6
max CK MB	35.5 ± 20.7
max Troponin	28.0 (21.7–37.3)
perioperative myocardial infarction	2 (0.64%)

Table 3. Cont.

Parameter	n (%)
stroke	0
new onset dialysis	0
postoperative angiography	2 (6.4%)
postoperative LAD intervention, graft occlusion	1 (0.3%)
re-exploration for bleeding	4 (1.3%)
blood transfusion in the ICU, Units	0.0 (0–4.0)

AF—atrial fibrillation, CK—creatine kinase, ICU—intensive care unit, and LAD—left descending artery.

The mean follow-up time was 16.3 ± 6.3 years. In-hospital mortality was 0.64% (n = 2), 6-month mortality was 0.97% (n = 3), and 1-year mortality was 0.97% (n = 3). We report a 5-year and 10-year mortality of 1.3% and 5.7%. Kaplan–Meier curve portrays the overall survival of our cohort (Figure 1).

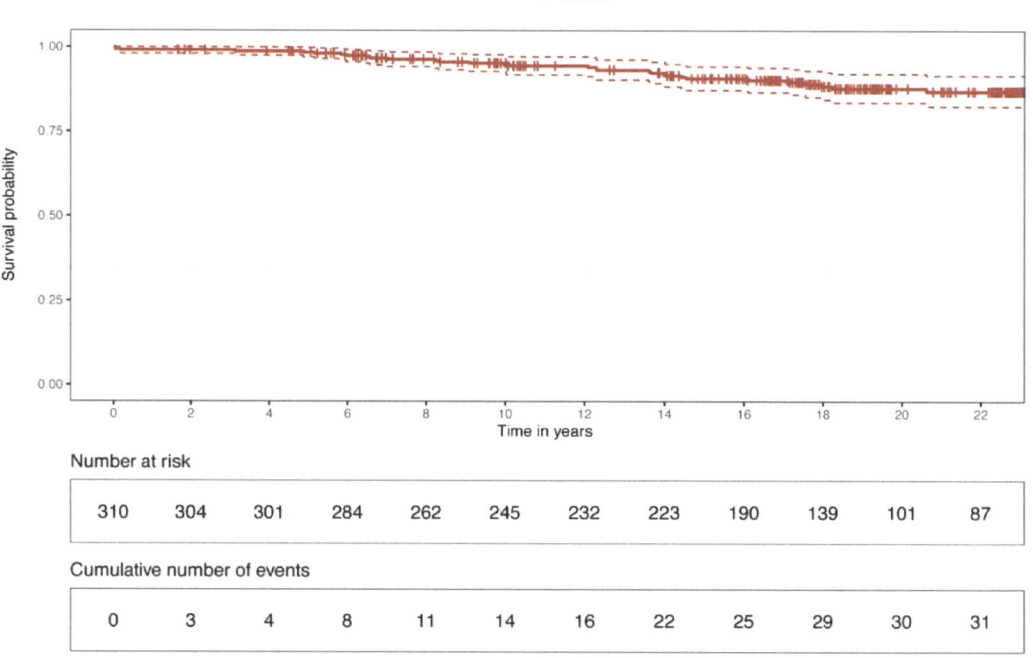

Figure 1. Overall survival.

The causes of death during the follow-up period are expressed in Table 4.

Table 4. Follow-up data.

Parameter	n (%)
Follow-up time, years	16.3 ± 6.3
in-hospital mortality	2 (0.64%)
6-months mortality	3 (0.97%)
1-year mortality	3 (0.97%)
5-year mortality	1.3%
10-year mortality	5.7%

Table 4. *Cont.*

Parameter	n (%)
Death at follow-up	31 (10%)
cardiac cause of death	6 (1.9%)
neurological cause of death	7 (2.3%)
oncological cause of death	8 (2.6%)
other cause of death	10 (3.2%)
coronary angiography	63 (20.3%)
bypass closure	5 (1.6%)

During the follow-up period, 63 patients (20.3%) underwent a diagnostic coronary angiography. In five patients (1.6%), LIMA-LAD bypass was not patent (after 4, 5 (×2), 7, and 18 years postoperatively).

4. Discussion

In recent years, MIDCAB surgery presented promising results as an effective and safe minimally invasive approach for coronary revascularization [4,6,7]. The less invasive nature of this approach provides advantages for various patient groups, including those with comorbidities that make a standard sternotomy impractical [5,7]. The present single-center, retrospective study reports our results on long-term survival and postoperative results of consecutive patients who underwent MIDCAB revascularization in our institution between July 1999 and April 2022. Our results further support that MIDCAB revascularization is an effective and safe strategy.

The mean operation time in our cohort was 129.7 ± 35.3, which is lower than the previously reported data [8,9]. The present study reports comparable short-term results with respect to the literature with an in-hospital mortality of 0.64%, a 6-month mortality of 0.97%, and a 1-year mortality of 0.97%. The mean follow-up time in the present study was 16.3 ± 6.3 years, which was longer than most of the comparable studies [7–11]. Our results regarding the 10-year survival rate (94.3%) for the entire cohort are favorable compared to the existing evidence in the literature [7,12–14].

Previously published studies reported comparable stroke and myocardial infarction (MI) rates between conventional CABG and minimally invasive approaches verifying its safety [15]. In line with previous evidence [8,10,16], our study reports no cases of perioperative stroke, no cases of new-onset dialysis, and only two cases (0.64%) of perioperative MI. In our study, we present seven cases (2.3%) of newly manifested AF, which is favorable compared to previously reported rates [8,16]. We report no need for intraoperative blood transfusion in our cohort and a short duration of ICU (1.0, 0–1.0 days) and in-hospital stay (8.7 ± 5.5 days), which is comparable to previously published data [8,9] reporting a significantly lower proportion of transfused patients and a shorter ICU and in-hospital stay amongst MIDCAB patients [16–18]. The conversion rate to sternotomy (3 cases, 1%), as well as the conversion to cardiopulmonary bypass (3 cases, 1%), was low and comparable to the evidence in the literature [10,12]. Four patients (1.3%) had to be re-explored for bleeding, a rate which is in line with previously published data [7,10,19].

The literature contains extensive debate about the long-term outcomes of MIDCAB compared to other minimally invasive coronary revascularization methods, such as percutaneous coronary intervention (PCI). For patients with multivessel coronary artery disease, evidence suggests that coronary artery bypass grafting offers more favorable outcomes than both medical therapy and PCI. Specifically, medical therapy has been associated with a higher occurrence of subsequent myocardial infarctions, increased need for additional revascularizations, and a higher incidence of cardiac death. Meanwhile, PCI is linked to a greater incidence of myocardial infarctions, an increased requirement for further revascularization, and a 1.46-fold increased risk of combined adverse events compared to CABG [20].

Several studies have shown similar rates of death, myocardial infarction, and stroke amongst PCI patients compared to MIDCAB, albeit with a notably higher rate of repeat revascularization in PCI patients [21–23]. A study by Merkle et al. has shown that although MIDCAB operation is linked to a longer ICU and hospital stay, it is associated with notably reduced occurrences of repeat revascularization and lower mortality rates compared to PCI [24].

Recent meta-analyses have highlighted the long-term advantages of MIDCAB over percutaneous coronary intervention. Specifically, studies have indicated that MIDCAB patients experience lower all-cause mortality and reduced rates of repeat revascularization compared to those undergoing PCI [25]. These findings align with earlier meta-analyses demonstrating that MIDCAB not only minimizes the need for subsequent interventions but also achieves comparable mortality rates and incidences of major adverse cardiac and cerebrovascular events to those of drug-eluting stents [26]. Additionally, when comparing minimally invasive left internal thoracic artery bypass to percutaneous transluminal coronary artery stenting for isolated left anterior descending artery lesions, MIDCAB has been shown to lead to fewer mid-term complications, further validating its efficacy and safety [27].

Research has extensively compared the safety and efficacy of the MIDCAB approach with both standard on-pump CABG and sternotomy off-pump CABG (OPCAB) [28]. Notably, a case-matched study by Lapierre et al. demonstrated that MIDCAB led to shorter hospital stays and quicker postoperative recovery compared to OPCAB [29]. This approach is also associated with several other benefits, including lower rates of blood transfusions and wound infections, due to the preservation of sternum integrity [30]. Although the study of Raja et al. further supported the safety of MIDCAB on a mean follow-up of 12.95 ± 0.47 years, it failed to prove its superiority compared to standard CABG [5].

As previously mentioned, our center has recently begun using the new Multistation^{TM} retractor (LSI Solutions, USA) in patients undergoing minimally invasive coronary revascularization. This innovative tool enhances surgical exposure and access, facilitating the harvesting of both the left and right internal mammary arteries (LIMA and RIMA) and allowing for complex multivessel revascularizations through smaller incisions. The Retro-Sterno^{TM} paddle, which is placed through a small 1.5 cm subxyphoidal incision, provides easier access to the RIMA through the left anterolateral thoracotomy, allowing its harvesting both under direct vision or endoscopically.

Current evidence on the MIDCAB approach is somewhat limited due to a scarcity of large prospective studies and randomized controlled trials, as well as variations in the definitions of techniques and complications, coupled with suboptimal clinical follow-up protocols [31]. Further studies are needed to better investigate the postoperative results of MIDCAB surgery and its benefits compared to other coronary revascularization approaches.

Due to the demanding learning curve associated with the MIDCAB approach [32,33], it is important to note that maintaining a high quality of the MIDCAB procedure is achievable when it is carried out in high-volume centers, enabling surgeons to effectively sustain their skills [12,32,34].

Limitations

This study presents limitations mainly related to its retrospective, observational, and single-center design.

The population of the present study comprises patients with diverse disease severity, ranging from single to multivessel coronary disease while also including mostly elective as well as a few emergent cases, which may affect the long-term survival and complication rates. It should also be mentioned that the patient cohort of the present study included a selected group of relatively low-risk patients and favorable baseline patient characteristics, thus the reported results should not be generalized to all with coronary artery disease. Moreover, our cohort presents the entire experience of our center also including the first cases. Taking into consideration the initial learning curve associated with the implementation of every new interventional technique may have impacted our results.

5. Conclusions

MIDCAB offers a viable and effective option for surgical myocardial revascularization with favorable long-term outcomes and minimal perioperative complications, particularly in low-risk patients. Our findings support the efficacy and safety of MIDCAB, suggesting its broader adoption in suitable candidates within high-volume centers. Further research is needed to validate these findings through prospective, multi-center trials to overcome limitations associated with retrospective analyses.

Author Contributions: A.Z. and A.W. conceptualized and designed this study; L.A., E.B., M.S. and A.S.M. provided statistical analysis and figures. All authors contributed to the acquisition, analysis, and interpretation of these data. All authors have read and agreed to the published version of the manuscript.

Funding: This research received no external funding.

Institutional Review Board Statement: The study was conducted in accordance with the Declaration of Helsinki. Ethical approval was granted by the Medical School of Hannover's Institutional Review Board (Nr. 11333_BO_K_2024, 4 April 2024).

Informed Consent Statement: Informed written consent was obtained from all participants, guaranteeing the confidentiality and anonymity of their data throughout the analysis.

Data Availability Statement: The data are available from the corresponding author upon reasonable request.

Conflicts of Interest: The authors declare no conflicts of interest.

References

1. Jha, A.K.; Fisher, E.S.; Li, Z.; Orav, E.J.; Epstein, A.M. Racial trends in the use of major procedures among the elderly. *N. Engl. J. Med.* **2005**, *353*, 683–691. [CrossRef] [PubMed]
2. Head, S.J.; Milojevic, M.; Taggart, D.P.; Puskas, J.D. Current Practice of State-of-the-Art Surgical Coronary Revascularization. *Circulation* **2017**, *136*, 1331–1345. [CrossRef] [PubMed]
3. Zubarevich, A.; Beltsios, E.T.; Arjomandi Rad, A.; Amanov, L.; Szczechowicz, M.; Ruhparwar, A.; Weymann, A. Sutureless Aortic Valve Prosthesis in Redo Procedures: Single-Center Experience. *Medicina* **2023**, *59*, 1126. [CrossRef] [PubMed]
4. Harky, A.; Chaplin, G.; Chan, J.S.K.; Eriksen, P.; MacCarthy-Ofosu, B.; Theologou, T.; Muir, A.D. The Future of Open Heart Surgery in the Era of Robotic and Minimal Surgical Interventions. *Heart Lung Circ.* **2020**, *29*, 49–61. [CrossRef] [PubMed]
5. Raja, S.G.; Garg, S.; Rochon, M.; Daley, S.; Robertis, F.D.; Bahrami, T. Short-term clinical outcomes and long-term survival of minimally invasive direct coronary artery bypass grafting. *Ann. Cardiothorac. Surg.* **2018**, *7*, 621. [CrossRef] [PubMed]
6. Van Praet, K.M.; Kofler, M.; Shafti, T.Z.N.; El Al, A.A.; van Kampen, A.; Amabile, A.; Torregrossa, G.; Kempfert, J.; Falk, V.; Balkhy, H.H.; et al. Minimally Invasive Coronary Revascularisation Surgery: A Focused Review of the Available Literature. *Interv. Cardiol.* **2021**, *16*, e08. [CrossRef] [PubMed]
7. Manuel, L.; Fong, L.S.; Betts, K.; Bassin, L.; Wolfenden, H. LIMA to LAD grafting returns patient survival to age-matched population: 20-year outcomes of MIDCAB surgery. *Interdiscip. Cardiovasc. Thorac. Surg.* **2022**, *35*, ivac243. [CrossRef] [PubMed]
8. Reuthebuch, O.; Stein, A.; Koechlin, L.; Gahl, B.; Berdajs, D.; Santer, D.; Eckstein, F. Five-Year Survival of Patients Treated with Minimally Invasive Direct Coronary Artery Bypass (MIDCAB) Compared with the General Swiss Population. *Thorac. Cardiovasc. Surg.* **2023**. *Epub ahead of print.* [CrossRef]
9. Seo, D.H.; Kim, J.S.; Park, K.H.; Lim, C.; Chung, S.R.; Kim, D.J. Mid-Term Results of Minimally Invasive Direct Coronary Artery Bypass Grafting. *Korean J. Thorac. Cardiovasc. Surg.* **2018**, *51*, 8–14. [CrossRef] [PubMed]
10. Reser, D.; van Hemelrijck, M.; Pavicevic, J.; Tolboom, H.; Holubec, T.; Falk, V.; Jacobs, S. Mid-Term Outcomes of Minimally Invasive Direct Coronary Artery Bypass Grafting. *Thorac. Cardiovasc. Surg.* **2015**, *63*, 313–318. [CrossRef]
11. Calafiore, A.M.; Giammarco, G.D.; Teodori, G.; Bosco, G.; D'Annunzio, E.; Barsotti, A.; Maddestra, N.; Paloscia, L.; Vitolla, G.; Sciarra, A.; et al. Left anterior descending coronary artery grafting via left anterior small thoracotomy without cardiopulmonary bypass. *Ann. Thorac. Surg.* **1996**, *61*, 1658–1663; discussion 1664–1665. [CrossRef]

12. Holzhey, D.M.; Cornely, J.P.; Rastan, A.J.; Davierwala, P.; Mohr, F.W. Review of a 13-year single-center experience with minimally invasive direct coronary artery bypass as the primary surgical treatment of coronary artery disease. *Heart Surg. Forum.* **2012**, *15*, E61–E68. [CrossRef] [PubMed]
13. Davierwala, P.M.; Verevkin, A.; Bergien, L.; von Aspern, K.; Deo, S.V.; Misfeld, M.; Holzhey, D.; Borger, M.A. Twenty-year outcomes of minimally invasive direct coronary artery bypass surgery: The Leipzig experience. *J. Thorac. Cardiovasc. Surg.* **2023**, *165*, 115–127.e4. [CrossRef] [PubMed]
14. Repossini, A.; Di Bacco, L.; Nicoli, F.; Passaretti, B.; Stara, A.; Jonida, B.; Muneretto, C. Minimally invasive coronary artery bypass: Twenty-year experience. *J. Thorac. Cardiovasc. Surg.* **2019**, *158*, 127–138.e1. [CrossRef] [PubMed]
15. Hammal, F.; Nagase, F.; Menon, D.; Ali, I.; Nagendran, J.; Stafinski, T. Robot-assisted coronary artery bypass surgery: A systematic review and meta-analysis of comparative studies. *Can. J. Surg.* **2020**, *63*, E491–E508. [CrossRef] [PubMed]
16. Ling, Y.; Bao, L.; Yang, W.; Chen, Y.; Gao, Q. Minimally invasive direct coronary artery bypass grafting with an improved rib spreader and a new-shaped cardiac stabilizer: Results of 200 consecutive cases in a single institution. *BMC Cardiovasc. Disord.* **2016**, *16*, 42. [CrossRef] [PubMed]
17. Zaouter, C.; Imbault, J.; Labrousse, L.; Abdelmoumen, Y.; Coiffic, A.; Colonna, G.; Jansens, J.L.; Ouattara, A. Association of Robotic Totally Endoscopic Coronary Artery Bypass Graft Surgery Associated with a Preliminary Cardiac Enhanced Recovery After Surgery Program: A Retrospective Analysis. *J. Cardiothorac. Vasc. Anesth.* **2015**, *29*, 1489–1497. [CrossRef] [PubMed]
18. Subramanian, V.A.; Patel, N.U. Current status of MIDCAB procedure. *Curr. Opin. Cardiol.* **2001**, *16*, 268–270. [CrossRef] [PubMed]
19. Al-Mulla, A.W.; Sarhan, H.H.T.; Abdalghafoor, T.; Al-Balushi, S.; El Kahlout, M.I.; Tbishat, L.; Alwaheidi, D.F.; Maksoud, M.; Omar, A.S.; Ashraf, S.; et al. Robotic Coronary Revascularization is Feasible and Safe: 10-year Single-Center Experience. *Heart Views* **2022**, *23*, 195–200. [PubMed]
20. Hueb, W.; Lopes, N.; Gersh, B.J.; Soares, P.R.; Ribeiro, E.E.; Pereira, A.C.; Favarato, D.; Rocha, A.S.; Hueb, A.C.; Ramires, J.A. Ten-year follow-up survival of the Medicine, Angioplasty, or Surgery Study (MASS II): A randomized controlled clinical trial of 3 therapeutic strategies for multivessel coronary artery disease. *Circulation* **2010**, *122*, 949–957. [CrossRef]
21. Blazek, S.; Rossbach, C.; Borger, M.A.; Fuernau, G.; Desch, S.; Eitel, I.; Stiermaier, T.; Lurz, P.; Holzhey, D.; Schuler, G.; et al. Comparison of sirolimus-eluting stenting with minimally invasive bypass surgery for stenosis of the left anterior descending coronary artery: 7-year follow-up of a randomized trial. *JACC Cardiovasc. Interv.* **2015**, *8 Pt A*, 30–38. [CrossRef]
22. Blazek, S.; Holzhey, D.; Jungert, C.; Borger, M.A.; Fuernau, G.; Desch, S.; Eitel, I.; de Waha, S.; Lurz, P.; Schuler, G.; et al. Comparison of bare-metal stenting with minimally invasive bypass surgery for stenosis of the left anterior descending coronary artery: 10-year follow-up of a randomized trial. *JACC Cardiovasc. Interv.* **2013**, *6*, 20–26. [CrossRef] [PubMed]
23. Jaffery, Z.; Kowalski, M.; Weaver, W.D.; Khanal, S. A meta-analysis of randomized control trials comparing minimally invasive direct coronary bypass grafting versus percutaneous coronary intervention for stenosis of the proximal left anterior descending artery. *Eur. J. Cardiothorac. Surg.* **2007**, *31*, 691–697. [CrossRef] [PubMed]
24. Merkle, J.; Zeriouh, M.; Sabashnikov, A.; Azizov, F.; Hohmann, C.; Weber, C.; Eghbalzadeh, K.; Said, Y.; Wahlers, T.; Michels, G. Minimally invasive direct coronary artery bypass graft surgery versus percutaneous coronary intervention of the LAD: Costs and long-term outcome. *Perfusion* **2019**, *34*, 323–329. [CrossRef] [PubMed]
25. Gianoli, M.; de Jong, A.R.; Jacob, K.A.; Namba, H.F.; van der Kaaij, N.P.; van der Harst, P.; Suyker, W.J.L. Minimally invasive surgery or stenting for left anterior descending artery disease—Meta-analysis. *Int. J. Cardiol. Heart Vasc.* **2022**, *40*, 101046. [CrossRef] [PubMed]
26. Raja, S.G.; Uzzaman, M.; Garg, S.; Santhirakumaran, G.; Lee, M.; Soni, M.K.; Khan, H. Comparison of minimally invasive direct coronary artery bypass and drug-eluting stents for management of isolated left anterior descending artery disease: A systematic review and meta-analysis of 7710 patients. *Ann. Cardiothorac. Surg.* **2018**, *7*, 567–576. [CrossRef] [PubMed]
27. Aziz, O.; Rao, C.; Panesar, S.S.; Jones, C.; Morris, S.; Darzi, A.; Athanasiou, T. Meta-analysis of minimally invasive internal thoracic artery bypass versus percutaneous revascularisation for isolated lesions of the left anterior descending artery. *BMJ* **2007**, *334*, 617. [CrossRef] [PubMed]
28. Xu, Y.; Li, Y.; Bao, W.; Qiu, S. MIDCAB versus off-pump CABG: Comparative study. *Hellenic. J. Cardiol.* **2020**, *61*, 120–124. [CrossRef] [PubMed]
29. Lapierre, H.; Chan, V.; Sohmer, B.; Mesana, T.G.; Ruel, M. Minimally invasive coronary artery bypass grafting via a small thoracotomy versus off-pump: A case-matched study. *Eur. J. Cardiothorac. Surg.* **2011**, *40*, 804–810. [CrossRef] [PubMed]
30. Ruel, M.; Une, D.; Bonatti, J.; McGinn, J.T. Minimally invasive coronary artery bypass grafting: Is it time for the robot? *Curr. Opin. Cardiol.* **2013**, *28*, 639–645. [CrossRef] [PubMed]
31. Cao, C.; Indraratna, P.; Doyle, M.; Tian, D.H.; Liou, K.; Munkholm-Larsen, S.; Uys, C.; Virk, S. A systematic review on robotic coronary artery bypass graft surgery. *Ann. Cardiothorac. Surg.* **2016**, *5*, 530–543. [CrossRef] [PubMed]
32. Okawa, Y.; Baba, H.; Hashimoto, M.; Tanaka, T.; Toyama, M.; Matsumoto, K.; Azuma, K. Comparison of standard coronary artery bypass grafting and minimary invasive direct coronary artery bypass grafting. Early and mid-term result. *Jpn J. Thorac. Cardiovasc. Surg.* **2000**, *48*, 725–729. [CrossRef] [PubMed]

33. Fatehi Hassanabad, A.; Kang, J.; Maitland, A.; Adams, C.; Kent, W.D.T. Review of Contemporary Techniques for Minimally Invasive Coronary Revascularization. *Innovations* **2021**, *16*, 231–243. [CrossRef] [PubMed]
34. Holzhey, D.M.; Jacobs, S.; Mochalski, M.; Walther, T.; Thiele, H.; Mohr, F.W.; Falk, V. Seven-year follow-up after minimally invasive direct coronary artery bypass: Experience with more than 1300 patients. *Ann. Thorac. Surg.* **2007**, *83*, 108–114. [CrossRef] [PubMed]

Disclaimer/Publisher's Note: The statements, opinions and data contained in all publications are solely those of the individual author(s) and contributor(s) and not of MDPI and/or the editor(s). MDPI and/or the editor(s) disclaim responsibility for any injury to people or property resulting from any ideas, methods, instructions or products referred to in the content.

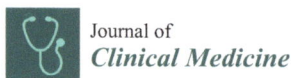 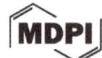

Article

Minimally Invasive Approach for Replacement of the Ascending Aorta towards the Proximal Aortic Arch

Florian Helms [1,*,†], Ezin Deniz [1,†], Heike Krüger [1], Alina Zubarevich [1], Jan Dieter Schmitto [1], Reza Poyanmehr [1], Martin Hinteregger [1], Andreas Martens [2], Alexander Weymann [1], Arjang Ruhparwar [1], Bastian Schmack [1,‡] and Aron-Frederik Popov [1,‡]

1. Division for Cardiothoracic-, Transplantation- and Vascular Surgery, Hannover Medical School, Carl-Neuberg-Str. 1, 30625 Hannover, Germany
2. Clinic for Cardiac Surgery, University Clinic Oldenburg, 26129 Oldenburg, Germany
* Correspondence: helms.florian@mh-hannover.de; Tel.: +49-511-532-1454; Fax: +49-511-532-8797
† These authors contributed equally to this work.
‡ These authors also contributed equally to this work.

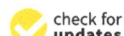

Abstract: Objectives: In recent years, minimally invasive approaches have been used with increasing frequency, even for more complex aortic procedures. However, evidence on the practicability and safety of expanding minimally invasive techniques from isolated operations of the ascending aorta towards more complex operations such as the hemiarch replacement is still scarce to date. **Methods:** A total of 86 patients undergoing elective surgical replacement of the ascending aorta with (n = 40) or without (n = 46) concomitant proximal aortic arch replacement between 2009 and 2023 were analyzed in a retrospective single-center analysis. Groups were compared regarding operation times, intra- and postoperative complications and long-term survival. **Results:** Operation times and ventilation times were significantly longer in the hemiarch replacement group. Despite this, no statistically significant differences between the two groups were observed for the duration of the ICU and hospital stay and postoperative complication rates. At ten-year follow-up, overall survival was 82.6% after isolated ascending aorta replacement and 86.3% after hemiarch replacement (p = 0.441). **Conclusions:** Expanding the indication for minimally invasive aortic surgery towards the proximal aortic arch resulted in comparable postoperative complication rates, length of hospital stay and overall long-term survival compared to the well-established minimally invasive isolated supracommissural ascending aorta replacement.

Keywords: minimally invasive surgery; aortic surgery; ascending aorta replacement; proximal aortic arch replacement; hemiarch replacement

Citation: Helms, F.; Deniz, E.; Krüger, H.; Zubarevich, A.; Schmitto, J.D.; Poyanmehr, R.; Hinteregger, M.; Martens, A.; Weymann, A.; Ruhparwar, A.; et al. Minimally Invasive Approach for Replacement of the Ascending Aorta towards the Proximal Aortic Arch. *J. Clin. Med.* **2024**, *13*, 3274. https://doi.org/10.3390/jcm13113274

Academic Editors: Manuel Wilbring and Emmanuel Andrès

Received: 26 April 2024
Revised: 24 May 2024
Accepted: 28 May 2024
Published: 31 May 2024

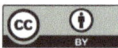

Copyright: © 2024 by the authors. Licensee MDPI, Basel, Switzerland. This article is an open access article distributed under the terms and conditions of the Creative Commons Attribution (CC BY) license (https://creativecommons.org/licenses/by/4.0/).

1. Introduction

Over the last two decades, minimally invasive techniques have developed rapidly in cardiac surgery, and the feasibility and safety of minimally invasive cardiac surgery have been demonstrated for different cardiac procedures [1,2]. Likewise, minimally invasive approaches have gained immense importance in aortic surgery as well and have become the standard approach for limited operations of the aortic valve, aortic root and ascending aorta in many centers [3–7]. For this, numerous techniques have been developed including different types of upper hemisternotomies as well as sternal sparing thoracotomy approaches [8–14]. Currently used surgical techniques and outcomes for minimally invasive surgery of the ascending aorta have been described in detail in a recent review from our working group [3]. In matched analyses, comparable results regarding safety outcomes, mortality and hospital stay have been reported for minimally invasive aortic root and ascending aorta replacement compared to the standard full sternotomy techniques [8,9,12]. In a recent study, Angerer et al. reported longer operation times but no differences in hospital stay or long-term outcome in minimally invasive ascending aorta replacement compared to full sternotomy [15]. Following this development, the minimally invasive approach has been continuously expanded to address more complex aortic pathologies through limited access sites. As one of these techniques, surgical repair of more distal parts of the ascending aorta and proximal aortic arch via upper hemisternotomies is now performed with increasing frequency [16]. In the current literature, this technique is also referred to as 'hemiarch replacement' [17]. However, including replacement of the proximal aortic arch in the repair distinctively increases the complexity of the operation compared to isolated replacement of the ascending aorta alone. Since cross-clamping of the ascending aorta proximal to the brachiocephalic trunk is not feasible for proximal aortic arch replacement, hypothermic circulatory arrest is generally inevitable and selective cerebral perfusion has to be established through minimally invasive access, which can be challenging depending on the cannulation strategy and access technique [3,9,10].

Consequently, while the results of the now well-established minimally invasive procedure to replace the aortic root and proximal ascending aorta are promising [7,8], further clinical evidence is needed regarding the significantly more complex procedure of additional proximal aortic arch replacement. We here report a 15-year single-center experience of expanding the minimally invasive approach towards the proximal aortic arch compared to the well-established minimally invasive technique for isolated supracommissural ascending aorta replacement.

2. Patients and Methods

2.1. Patients

Between June 2009 and May 2023, 86 consecutive patients underwent elective minimally invasive ascending aorta replacement with or without concomitant proximal aortic arch replacement at our tertiary care center. Patient data including preoperative characteristics, intraoperative and postoperative course and complications as well as long-term postoperative survival were collected prospectively in our institutional database and analyzed retrospectively for this study. Postoperative follow-up was performed during regular visits in our outpatient clinic. Patients requiring concomitant aortic root or aortic valve surgery were excluded from the study. The necessity for concomitant procedures of the atrioventricular valves or coronary bypass grafting as well as emergency situations and redo operations contraindicate the upper hemisternotomy approach in our institution.

2.2. Study Design and Variables

For a retrospective single-center analysis, the study population was divided into two groups. The first group included all patients who received isolated minimally invasive ascending aorta replacement, while the second group consisted of patients in which additional proximal aortic arch repair was performed. For sorting into the groups, the following definitions were used: isolated ascending aorta replacement was defined as implantation of a straight aortic graft with a proximal suture line positioned on or above the sinotubular junction and a distal suture line located proximal to the brachiocephalic trunk within the Ishimaru zone 0, facilitating continuous cross-clamping of the distal ascending aorta and continuous body perfusion via direct aortic cannulation. In contrast, the distal suture line of proximal aortic arch replacement was placed more distally between zone 0 in the outer curvature and zone 1 in the inner curvature of the aortic arch to facilitate narrowing of the proximal arch while avoiding reimplantation of the brachiocephalic trunk. In these cases of hemiarch replacement, an open distal anastomosis is necessary, requiring hypothermic circulatory arrest.

For this study, preexisting coronary artery disease was defined as any treated or untreated flow-limiting coronary artery obstruction diagnosed by coronary angiography. Chronic kidney disease was defined as a decreased glomerular filtration rate of less than 60 mL/min (1.73 m^2) for at least 3 months [18]. Any prior surgical procedures involving the heart or large intrathoracic vessels were summarized as cardiac preoperations. Chronic type A aortic dissection was defined as any aortic dissection involving the ascending aorta persisting for more than 14 days after the initial intima rupture [19].

2.3. Surgical Techniques

For both isolated ascending aorta replacement and hemiarch replacement, an upper J-shaped hemisternotomy to the third or fourth intercostal space was used. After applying the sternal retractor, pericardial stay sutures were placed to enhance exposure, and heparinization with a dose of 400–500 IU/kgBWT (body weight) was initiated. After reaching an activated clotting time of >400 s, distal ascending aortic and direct right atrial cannulation were performed in standard fashion. Venting was established through the main pulmonary artery in this minimally invasive setting. Continuous carbon dioxide insufflation was initiated, extracorporeal circulation was started, the aorta was cross-clamped, and cold blood cardioplegia was administered. For hemiarch replacement, cooling was initiated with a target bladder temperature of 25 °C. The aorta was opened and resected proximally until directly above the sinotubular junction. For isolated supracommissural ascending aorta replacement, Terumo Aortic Gelweave® (Terumo Aortic, Inchinnan, UK) straight aortic grafts were used, and distal and proximal anastomoses were made using running Prolene® sutures (Prolene, Somerville, NJ, USA). For additional hemiarch replacement, the Terumo Aortic Gelweave Anteflo® aortic grafts were used. The decision for or against selective cerebral perfusion was based on the expected circulatory arrest time taking into consideration anatomical features including accessibility of the distal anastomosis site and quality of the aortic tissue. If necessary, antegrade cerebral perfusion via direct cannulation of the brachiocephalic trunk ($n = 15$) or retrograde cerebral perfusion via the superior vena cava ($n = 5$) was performed. For expected circulatory arrest times of less than 10 min, no selective cerebral perfusion was used ($n = 20$). The distal anastomosis for hemiarch replacement was performed in an oblique fashion reaching from zone 0 in the outer curvature to zone 1 in the inner curvature. After this, the arterial line of the extracorporeal circulation was placed in the side branch of the Anteflo® prosthesis (Terumo Aortic, Inchinnan, UK), and extracorporeal circulation was continued. Subsequently, the proximal prosthesio-aortic anastomosis at the level of the sinotubular junction was performed. After careful deairing, the patients were weaned from extracorporeal circulation in standard fashion in both groups.

2.4. Statistical Analysis

IBM SPSS Statistics 28 (IBM Corp., Armonk, NY, USA, 1989, 2021) was used for statistical analyses. The Kolmogorov–Smirnov test was used to test for normal distribution, and normally distributed data are given as mean and standard deviation (SD). Median and interquartile range (Q1–Q3) are used to present non-normally distributed data. Homoscedasticity was tested using the Lavene test. The T-test or the Mann–Whitney test were used to compare continuous variables. Categorial variables are shown as total numbers (n) and percentages. The Kaplan–Meier survival estimates including the log-rank test were used to analyze survival. Differences were considered significant at $p < 0.05$.

3. Results

Proximal aortic arch replacement was performed in 40 (46.5%) of 86 patients included in this study. With a median patient age of 69 years (IQR 64.4–75.4 years) vs. 64.5 (IQR 53.5–74.4, $p = 0.029$), patients in the hemiarch group were slightly older compared to the isolated ascending aorta replacement group. Likewise, they more often had a positive history of preexisting coronary artery disease, while bicuspid aortic valve morphology was distinctively more frequent in patients undergoing isolated ascending aorta replacement (23.5% vs. 7.5%, $p = 0.04$) (Table 1). While the indication for surgery in the vast majority of patients in both groups was aortic aneurysm, each case of penetrating aortic ulcer and chronic type A aortic dissection was present in the group that underwent proximal aortic arch replacement.

Table 1. Preoperative characteristics. COPD = chronic obstructive pulmonary disease. Values in bold mark statistically significant differences with $p < 0.05$.

Characteristics	Ascending Aorta Replacement (n = 46)	Proximal Aortic Arch Replacement (n = 40)	p-Value
Sex (male)	22 (47.8%)	14 (35.0%)	0.229
Age (years)	64.5 (53.5–74.4)	69.0 (64.4–75.4)	**0.029**
Coronary artery disease	6 (13.0%)	14 (35.0%)	**0.016**
Atrial fibrillation	5 (10.9%)	4 (10.0%)	0.895
Pulmonary artery embolism	3 (6.5%)	1 (2.5%)	0.337
Persistent foramen ovale	2 (4.3%)	0 (0.0%)	0.182
Preoperative stroke	1 (2.2%)	3 (7.5%)	0.242
Diabetes	2 (4.3%)	2 (5.0%)	0.886
Chonic kidney disease	1 (2.2%)	3 (7.5%)	0.242
COPD	4 (8.7%)	4 (10.0%)	0.835
Bicuspid aortic valve	11 (23.5%)	3 (7.5%)	**0.040**
Aortitis	2 (4.3%)	1 (2.5%)	0.641
Chronic aortic dissection	0 (0.0%)	1 (2.5%)	0.281
Penetrating aortic ulcer	0 (0.0%)	1 (2.5%)	0.281
Cardiac preoperation	0 (0.0%)	1 (2.5%)	0.281

Operation time and bypass time were significantly longer in the hemiarch group. Here, the median hypothermic circulatory arrest time was 9.5 min (IQR 7.0–18.0 min). In one case (2–5%) in the hemiarch group, conversion to full sternotomy was necessary due to bleeding that was not controllable via the minimally invasive access point (Table 2).

Table 2. Intraoperative characteristics. Values in bold mark statistically significant differences with $p < 0.05$.

Characteristics	Ascending Aorta Replacement (n = 46)	Proximal Aortic Arch Replacement (n = 40)	p-Value
Concomitant cardiac procedure	3 (6.5%)	2 (5.0%)	0.764
Graft size (mm)	28 (26–30)	30 (28–30)	0.130
Operation time (min)	168 (143–204)	223 (207–243)	**<0.001**
Bypass time (min)	77 (65–102)	123 (104–139)	**<0.001**
Cross-clamp time (min)	47 (39–57)	51 (40–67)	0.301
Conversion to full sternotomy	0 (0.0%)	1 (2.5%)	0.281

In the early postoperative course, ventilation time after proximal aortic arch replacement was approximately twice as long as after isolated ascending aorta replacement (20.4 ± 7.0 vs. 10.3 ± 4.8 min, $p = 0.009$). Compared to that, the length of stay at the intensive care unit and postoperative hospital stay differed less distinctively and did not reach statistical significance (Table 3). Within the study population, no cases of postoperative dialysis requirement or paraplegia and paraparesis were found in both groups.

The survival analysis revealed one in-hospital death (2.2%) in the isolated ascending aorta replacement group as well as one death after discharge within the first postoperative month (2.5%) in the hemiarch group ($p = 0.920$ for 30-day mortality). Median follow-up time for long-term survival was 6.0 years. In the Kaplan–Meier analysis, no significant differences between the two groups were found with an overall survival of over 80% after 10 years of follow-up in both groups (log rank = 0.441) (Figure 1).

Table 3. Postoperative characteristics. ICU = intensive care unit. Values in bold mark statistically significant differences with $p < 0.05$.

Characteristics	Ascending Aorta Replacement (n = 46)	Proximal Aortic Arch Replacement (n = 40)	p-Value
Ventilation time (hours)	10.3 ± 4.8	20.4 ± 7.0	**0.009**
ICU stay (days)	2.02 ± 2.1	2.83 ± 2.8	0.134
Hospital stay (days)	8 (7–11)	10 (8–13)	0.111
Reanimation (ventricular fibrillation)	1 (2.2%)	2 (5.0%)	0.476
Delirium	0 (0.0%)	2 (5.0%)	0.125
Atrial fibrillation	6 (13.0%)	5 (12.5%)	0.940
Re-thoracotomy	0 (0.0%)	2 (5.0%)	0.125
Tracheotomy	0 (0.0%)	1 (2.5%)	0.281
Stroke	1 (2.2%)	3 (7.5%)	0.242

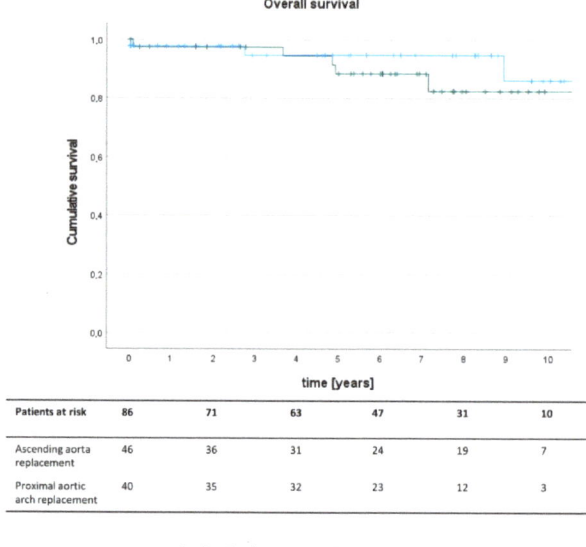

Figure 1. Kaplan–Meier analysis of long-term overall postoperative survival after isolated ascending aorta replacement (blue) or concomitant hemiarch replacement (green). Censored data are marked by horizontal lines.

4. Discussion

The main findings of this study can be summarized as follows: (1) Both isolated ascending aorta replacement and hemiarch replacement could be performed safely through a minimally invasive access site with a low conversion rate to full sternotomy. (2) Expanding the minimally invasive approach towards proximal aortic arch replacement prolonged the ventilation time but did not significantly increase the duration of the ICU or hospital stay. (3) In long-term follow-up, overall survival did not differ significantly between the two groups.

The safety and feasibility of minimally invasive ascending aorta replacement either alone or in combination with aortic valve or aortic root replacement has been demonstrated in different studies over the last few years [8,9,12,14]. In a propensity score-matched analysis of patients undergoing aortic valve replacement with supracommissural ascending aorta replacement via a minimally invasive partial sternotomy compared to classical full sternotomy, Haunschild et al. found similar results concerning safety and long-term durability outcomes [8]. They reported an in-hospital mortality of 1.7% in the minimal access group, which is within the range of our findings of an in-hospital mortality rate of 2.2% for the isolated ascending aorta replacement group and 1.2% for the entire study population. With these values, the early mortality after ascending aorta replacement in this study is similar to previously published mortality rates for minimally invasive approaches and within the range of the early mortality reported for ascending aorta replacement through full sternotomy [8,20].

However, the above-mentioned studies were mainly focused on the replacement of the proximal ascending aorta and did not involve hemiarch repair. Since replacement of the proximal aortic arch requires an open distal anastomosis, hypothermic circulatory arrest and not infrequently selective cerebral perfusion, first approaches for minimally invasive aortic surgery were limited to the proximal ascending aorta. In this field, a relatively broad basis of clinical evidence has been provided to date [3]. In contrast, chronologically later expansion of the minimally invasive technique towards the proximal has mainly been reported in the form of subgroup analyses with smaller case numbers among heterogeneous study populations to date: here, Kaneko et al. reported a 9-year single center experience of minimally invasive aortic valve and ascending aortic surgery [11]. Within their study cohort of 109 patients, 8 patients underwent concomitant proximal aortic arch replacement. In a combined subgroup analysis together with other concomitant procedures including Bentall or David operations, they reported an early mortality of 3.7% with no cases of conversion to full sternotomy. Although no specific subgroup analysis for proximal aortic arch replacement was performed by Kaneko et al. due to the limited number of cases, these results are consistent with our findings regarding postoperative complication rates. However, we saw one conversion to full sternotomy in our hemiarch study population. For long-term survival, they report a survival rate of approximately 80% after 10 years for their entire study population, which is comparable to the overall survival rate for both groups in the analysis presented here.

In another report by Deschka et al., 11 out of 50 patients undergoing minimally invasive surgery of the aortic root and ascending aorta received concomitant proximal aortic arch replacement [16]. While they report excellent short-term outcomes, they too report comparatively long postoperative ventilation periods with a mean ventilation time of 29 h. This observation is consistent with our findings of comparatively long postoperative ventilation times after proximal aortic arch replacement and may be due to prolonged warming periods after hypothermic circulatory arrest.

In a more recent propensity score-matched analysis including a total of 36 patients, Wu et al. compared minimally invasive techniques to classical full sternotomy for complex procedures in the setting of aortic dissection [21]. In addition to hemiarch replacement, their cohort also included 13 cases of total aortic arch replacement via upper hemisternotomy, which were performed using the arch-first technique, involving reconstruction of the supraaortic vessels prior to frozen elephant trunk implantation.

In this combined study population of different, more complex concomitant procedures, they found similar postoperative complication rates compared to isolated ascending aorta replacement or classical full sternotomy approaches; in-hospital mortality was overall low with one death recorded in the hemisternotomy group. Here, cross-clamp times were slightly longer in the hemisternotomy group. However, in their experience, the length of ICU stay and hospital stay were even shorter when using the minimally invasive approach. Our findings regarding the postoperative complication rates after hemiarch replacement confirm these reports. Compared to isolated ascending aorta replacement, performing proximal aortic arch replacement did not result in higher rates of postoperative complications or prolonged length of stay in our analysis.

5. Limitations and Conclusions

As this study is a retrospective single-center analysis, certain limitations need to be considered including a possible selection bias. Additionally, urgent and emergent cases were excluded from the analysis, and data obtained from the elective setting cannot be extrapolated to more urgent procedures. Additionally, minimally invasive proximal aortic arch replacement was not compared to hemiarch replacement via classical full sternotomy in this study. Lastly, minor differences between the study groups may not have been recorded or reached statistical significance due to the limited number of cases included in the study, which furthermore prohibited subgroup analyses of different age groups within the study population.

Expanding the indication for elective minimally invasive aortic surgery towards the proximal aortic arch resulted in comparable postoperative complication rates, length of hospital stay and overall long-term survival compared to the well-established minimally invasive isolated supracommissural ascending aorta replacement. This evidence suggests that even the more complex operation of hemiarch replacement requiring an open distal anastomosis and circulatory arrest can be performed safely through a minimally invasive access point with a similar outcome compared to isolated ascending aorta replacement.

Author Contributions: Conceptualization: A.M., A.-F.P., B.S., A.R., F.H. and E.D.; investigation: F.H., E.D. and H.K.; methodology: M.H., F.H. and E.D.; project administration: A.-F.P., B.S., J.D.S., M.H. and A.R.; resources: R.P., M.H. and H.K.; supervision: A.-F.P., B.S., A.Z., A.W., J.D.S. and B.S.; validation: A.-F.P., A.W., B.S., A.Z., F.H., E.D. and R.P.; visualization: F.H. and E.D.; writing—original draft: F.H. and E.D.; writing—review and editing: A.-F.P., B.S., F.H., J.D.S. and E.D. All authors have read and agreed to the published version of the manuscript.

Funding: This research did not receive external funding.

Institutional Review Board Statement: Ethical review and approval were waived for this study as it is a purely retrospective data analysis.

Informed Consent Statement: Informed consent was obtained from all subjects involved in the study.

Data Availability Statement: Data used in this study are available from the corresponding author upon request.

Conflicts of Interest: The authors declare no conflicts of interest.

References

1. Dieberg, G.; Smart, N.A.; King, N. Minimally invasive cardiac surgery: A systematic review and meta-analysis. *Int. J. Cardiol.* **2016**, *223*, 554–560. [CrossRef] [PubMed]
2. Claessens, J.; Rottiers, R.; Vandenbrande, J.; Gruyters, I.; Yilmaz, A.; Kaya, A.; Stessel, B. Quality of life in patients undergoing minimally invasive cardiac surgery: A systematic review. *Indian J. Thorac. Cardiovasc. Surg.* **2023**, *39*, 367–380. [CrossRef] [PubMed]
3. Helms, F.; Schmack, B.; Weymann, A.; Hanke, J.S.; Natanov, R.; Martens, A.; Ruhparwar, A.; Popov, A.-F. Expanding the Minimally Invasive Approach towards the Ascending Aorta-A Practical Overview of the Currently Available Techniques. *Medicina* **2023**, *59*, 1618. [CrossRef] [PubMed]
4. Jahangiri, M.; Hussain, A.; Akowuah, E. Minimally invasive surgical aortic valve replacement. *Heart* **2019**, *105* (Suppl. 2), s5–s10. [CrossRef] [PubMed]
5. Monsefi, N.; Risteski, P.; Miskovic, A.; Moritz, A.; Zierer, A. Midterm Results of a Minimally Invasive Approach in David Procedure. *Thorac. Cardiovasc. Surg.* **2018**, *66*, 301–306. [CrossRef] [PubMed]
6. Sun, L.; Zheng, J.; Chang, Q.; Tang, Y.; Feng, J.; Sun, X.; Zhu, X. Aortic root replacement by ministernotomy: Technique and potential benefit. *Ann. Thorac. Surg.* **2000**, *70*, 1958–1961. [CrossRef] [PubMed]
7. Shrestha, M.; Kaufeld, T.; Shrestha, P.; Martens, A.; Rustum, S.; Rudolph, L.; Krüger, H.; Arar, M.; Haverich, A.; Beckmann, E. Valve-sparing David procedure via minimally invasive access does not compromise outcome. *Front. Cardiovasc. Med.* **2022**, *9*, 966126. [CrossRef] [PubMed]

8. Haunschild, J.; van Kampen, A.; von Aspern, K.; Misfeld, M.; Davierwala, P.; Saeed, D.; Borger, M.A.; Etz, C.D. Supracommissural replacement of the ascending aorta and the aortic valve via partial versus full sternotomy-a propensity-matched comparison in a high-volume centre. *Eur. J. Cardiothorac. Surg.* **2022**, *61*, 479–487. [CrossRef] [PubMed]
9. Lamelas, J.; Chen, P.C.; Loor, G.; LaPietra, A. Successful Use of Sternal-Sparing Minimally Invasive Surgery for Proximal Ascending Aortic Pathology. *Ann. Thorac. Surg.* **2018**, *106*, 742–748. [CrossRef] [PubMed]
10. LaPietra, A.; Santana, O.; Pineda, A.M.; Mihos, C.G.; Lamelas, J. Outcomes of aortic valve and concomitant ascending aorta replacement performed via a minimally invasive right thoracotomy approach. *Innovations* **2014**, *9*, 339–342, discussion 342. [PubMed]
11. Kaneko, T.; Couper, G.S.; Borstlap, W.A.A.; Nauta, F.J.H.; Wollersheim, L.; McGurk, S.; Cohn, L.H. Minimal-access aortic valve replacement with concomitant aortic procedure: A 9-year experience. *Innovations* **2012**, *7*, 368–371. [PubMed]
12. Tabata, M.; Khalpey, Z.; Aranki, S.F.; Couper, G.S.; Cohn, L.H.; Shekar, P.S. Minimal access surgery of ascending and proximal arch of the aorta: A 9-year experience. *Ann. Thorac. Surg.* **2007**, *84*, 67–72. [CrossRef] [PubMed]
13. Svensson, L.G.; Nadolny, E.M.; Kimmel, W.A. Minimal access aortic surgery including re-operations. *Eur. J. Cardiothorac. Surg.* **2001**, *19*, 30–33. [CrossRef] [PubMed]
14. Byrne, J.G.; Karavas, A.N.; Cohn, L.H.; Adams, D.H. Minimal access aortic root, valve, and complex ascending aortic surgery. *Curr. Cardiol. Rep.* **2000**, *2*, 549–557. [CrossRef] [PubMed]
15. Angerer, M.; Pollari, F.; Hitzl, W.; Weber, L.; Sirch, J.; Fischlein, T. Isolated or Combined Ascending Aortic Replacement through a Partial Sternotomy: Early and Midterm Outcomes. *Thorac. Cardiovasc. Surg.* **2024**, 4–16, ahead of print.
16. Deschka, H.; Erler, S.; Machner, M.; El-Ayoubi, L.; Alken, A.; Wimmer-Greinecker, G. Surgery of the ascending aorta, root remodelling and aortic arch surgery with circulatory arrest through partial upper sternotomy: Results of 50 consecutive cases. *Eur. J. Cardiothorac. Surg.* **2013**, *43*, 580–584. [CrossRef] [PubMed]
17. El-Hamamsy, I.; Ouzounian, M.; Demers, P.; McClure, S.; Hassan, A.; Dagenais, F.; Chu, M.W.; Pozeg, Z.; Bozinovski, J.; Peterson, M.D.; et al. State-of-the-Art Surgical Management of Acute Type A Aortic Dissection. *Can. J. Cardiol.* **2016**, *32*, 100–109. [CrossRef] [PubMed]
18. Webster, A.C.; Nagler, E.V.; Morton, R.L.; Masson, P. Chronic Kidney Disease. *Lancet* **2017**, *389*, 1238–1252. [CrossRef] [PubMed]
19. Hynes, C.F.; Greenberg, M.D.; Sarin, S.; Trachiotis, G.D. Chronic Type A Aortic Dissection. *Aorta* **2016**, *4*, 16–21. [CrossRef] [PubMed]
20. Staromłyński, J.; Kowalewski, M.; Sarnowski, W.; Smoczyński, R.; Witkowska, A.; Bartczak, M.; Drobiński, D.; Wierzba, W.; Suwalski, P. Midterm results of less invasive approach to ascending aorta and aortic root surgery. *J. Thorac. Dis.* **2020**, *12*, 6446–6457. [CrossRef] [PubMed]
21. Wu, Y.; Jiang, W.; Li, D.; Chen, L.; Ye, W.; Ren, C.; Xiao, C. Surgery of ascending aorta with complex procedures for aortic dissection through upper mini-sternotomy versus conventional sternotomy. *J. Cardiothorac. Surg.* **2020**, *15*, 57. [CrossRef] [PubMed]

Disclaimer/Publisher's Note: The statements, opinions and data contained in all publications are solely those of the individual author(s) and contributor(s) and not of MDPI and/or the editor(s). MDPI and/or the editor(s) disclaim responsibility for any injury to people or property resulting from any ideas, methods, instructions or products referred to in the content.

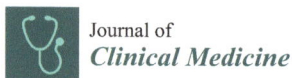
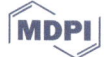

Article

Combined Minimally Invasive Mitral Valve Surgery and Percutaneous Coronary Intervention: A Hybrid Concept for Patients with Mitral Valve and Coronary Pathologies

Martín Moscoso-Ludueña [1,†], Maximilian Vondran [2,†], Marc Irqsusi [3], Holger Nef [4,5], Ardawan J. Rastan [1,3] and Tamer Ghazy [3,*]

1. Department of Cardiac and Vascular Surgery, Rotenburg Heart and Vascular Centre, 36199 Rotenburg an der Fulda, Germany; m.moscoso-luduena@hkz-rotenburg.de (M.M.-L.)
2. Department of Cardiac and Vascular Surgery, Klinikum Karlsburg, Heart and Diabetes Center Mecklenburg-Western Pommerania, 17495 Carlsburg, Germany; vondran.m@drguth.de
3. Department of Cardiac Surgery, Marburg University Hospital, Philipps University of Marburg, Baldingerstrasse, 35043 Marburg, Germany; irqsusi@med.uni-marburg.de
4. Department of Cardiology, Rotenburg Heart and Vascular Centre, 36199 Rotenburg an der Fulda, Germany
5. Department of Cardiology, Giessen University Hospital, 35392 Giessen, Germany
* Correspondence: tamer.ghazy@uk-gm.de; Tel.: +49-6421-5866223
† These authors contributed equally to this work.

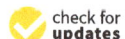

Citation: Moscoso-Ludueña, M.; Vondran, M.; Irqsusi, M.; Nef, H.; Rastan, A.J.; Ghazy, T. Combined Minimally Invasive Mitral Valve Surgery and Percutaneous Coronary Intervention: A Hybrid Concept for Patients with Mitral Valve and Coronary Pathologies. *J. Clin. Med.* **2023**, *12*, 5553. https://doi.org/10.3390/jcm12175553

Academic Editor: Francesco Formica

Received: 16 July 2023
Revised: 12 August 2023
Accepted: 16 August 2023
Published: 26 August 2023

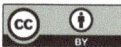

Copyright: © 2023 by the authors. Licensee MDPI, Basel, Switzerland. This article is an open access article distributed under the terms and conditions of the Creative Commons Attribution (CC BY) license (https:// creativecommons.org/licenses/by/ 4.0/).

Abstract: We evaluated the feasibility of hybrid percutaneous coronary intervention (PCI) and minimally invasive mitral valve surgery (MIMVS) in patients with concomitant coronary and mitral disease. Of 534 patients who underwent MIMVS at our institution between 2012 and 2018, those with combined mitral and single vessel coronary pathologies who underwent MIMVS and PCI were included. Patients were excluded if they had endocarditis or required emergency procedures. Preprocedural, procedural, and postprocedural data were retrospectively analyzed. In total, 10 patients (median age, 75 years; 7 males) with a median ejection fraction (EF) of 60% were included. Nine patients underwent PCI before and one after MIMVS. The success rate was 100% in both procedures. There were no postoperative myocardial infarctions or strokes. Two patients developed delirium and one required re-thoracotomy for bleeding. The median stay in intensive care and the hospital was 3 and 8 days, respectively. The 30-day survival rate was 100%. A hybrid PCI and MIMVS approach is feasible in patients with mitral valve and single vessel coronary disease. In combined pathologies, the revascularization strategy should be evaluated independent from the mitral valve pathology in the presence of MIMVS expertise. Extension of this recommendation to multivessel disease should be evaluated in future studies.

Keywords: mitral valve; minimally invasive; PCI; hybrid

1. Introduction

There is an increasing demand for minimally invasive mitral valve surgery (MIMVS) because of the cosmetic benefits, shorter hospital stay, and avoidance of sternotomy and its wound complications, making it a more desirable option than sternotomy. The aim of MIMVS is to treat patients with mitral valve pathologies using a favorable surgical approach [1,2]. However, the presence of a concomitant coronary pathology might influence the treatment strategy for both the coronary pathology and the mitral valve disease. According to the European Society of Cardiology (ESC) and the European Association of Cardiothoracic Surgery (EACTS) guidelines for myocardial revascularization, the choice of revascularization strategy (percutaneous coronary intervention [PCI] vs. coronary artery bypass grafting [CABG]) might be influenced by the presence of any indications of further cardiac procedures, such as valve surgery [3]. Based on these recommendations, patients with concomitant mitral valve and coronary pathologies—who are candidates for concomitant surgical revascularization according to the latest ESC/EACTS guidelines—are usually operated on via the median sternotomy to allow sufficient exposure of the coronary arteries [3].

The guidelines do not differentiate between single, double, or triple vessel disease in cases of concomitant valve surgery or between minimally invasive or classic approaches for valve therapy. Single vessel disease, which can be treated sufficiently endovascularly, is recommended to be treated surgically if concomitant valve surgery is to be performed [3]. Yet, this decision might be the leading indication for changing the surgical approach and denying the patient a minimally invasive procedure. The feasibility of MIMVS and PCI as a hybrid concept for patients with mitral valve and coronary pathologies is yet to be investigated. The aim of this study was to present our institution's initial experience with this hybrid concept in patients with combined pathologies.

2. Materials and Methods

2.1. Patient Cohort

Between January 2012 and April 2018, 534 patients who underwent isolated or combined MIMVS at our institution were screened for inclusion in this retrospective descriptive study. Patients were included if they had a combined mitral pathology and an indication for single vessel coronary revascularization and underwent hybrid therapy with MIMVS and interventional therapy for coronary disease. Patients who underwent a non-planned PCI or emergency procedures and those with endocarditis were excluded from the study. The study was approved by the institutional review board.

2.2. Data Collection

All data were collected from the patient records. The pre-management patient data, decision of the heart team, PCI, and operative procedural details as well as post-management results were retrospectively collected and analyzed.

2.3. Statistical Analysis and Reporting

Continuous variables are presented as medians with interquartile ranges (IQRs). Categorical variables are presented as absolute numbers. All statistical tests were performed using SPSS v22.0 (IBM Inc., Armonk, NY, USA).

3. Results

Overall, 10 patients who met the inclusion criteria were included in the analysis.

3.1. Demographic and Medical Data

Tables 1 and 2 summarizes the patient demographic and medical data. The overall median age was 75 years and seven patients were males. The median body mass index was 29.4 (23.7–31.6) kg/m^2. The comorbidities included hyperlipidemia ($n = 7$), renal insufficiency ($n = 4$), and diabetes mellitus ($n = 3$). The median creatinine value in the patient cohort was 1.08 mg/dl (0.84–1.87). None of the patients were on dialysis or had chronic obstructive pulmonary disease (COPD), liver failure, or peripheral vascular disease.

The analysis of the cardiac data revealed a median left ventricular ejection fraction (EF) of 60% (40–60%). Three patients had atrial fibrillation. All patients were of New York Heart Association (NYHA) class 3. Two patients were of Canadian Cardiac Society (CCS) class 2. All patients had mitral valve insufficiency with no stenosis and one patient had tricuspid regurgitation. None of the patients had aortic valve or aortic diseases. There were no cases of acute myocardial infarctions. Four patients had a past history of myocardial infarction; one patient each had it within 1 month and 90 days before the procedure, while two patients had it more than 90 days before the procedure. Two patients had a history of CABG in 1993 and 2003, respectively, both of whom underwent totally arterial bypass grafting to the left coronary system with no bypass grafting to the then non-diseased right coronary system that required intervention in the present study. Coronary angiography confirmed patent bypass grafts. None of the patients had a previous mitral valve surgery. The details of coronary findings are summarized in Table 1 and those of the mitral valve pathology are summarized in Table 2.

Table 1. Preoperative data.

Variables	Result
Demographic data	
Age, years (IQR)	75 (64–81)
Males, n	7
Body mass index, kg/m^2 (IQR)	29.4 (23.7–31.6)
Risk factors	
Arterial hypertension, n	9
Diabetes mellitus, n	3
Hyperlipidemia, n	7
History of smoking, n	1
Renal insufficiency, n	4
Previous cardiac surgery, n	2
EuroSCORE II, % (IQR)	8.1 (2.5–8.6)
STS score, % (IQR)	1.2 (0.7–3.1)
Cardiac data	
NYHA class, median	3
Mitral valve insufficiency, n	10
Ejection fraction, % (IQR)	60 (40–60)
Tricuspid valve insufficiency, n	1
Pulmonary hypertension >60 mmHg, n	0
History of myocardial infarction, n	4
Atrial fibrillation, n	3
Pacemaker/AICD, n	1
Coronary data	
Previously operated patients	
Patient No.1 CABG	LIMA to D1 and LAD, RIMA-T to M1, intact grafts
Patient No.2 CABG	LIMA to LAD, RIMA-T to M1, intact grafts
RCA as Target vessel for PCI	both patients
Previously non-operated patients	
RCA as Target vessel for PCI, n	1
LAD as Target vessel for PCI, n	3
D1 as Target vessel for PCI, n	1
RCX as Target vessel for PCI, n	3

Abbreviations: NYHA: New York Heart Association; AICD: automated implantable cardioverter defibrillator; CABG: coronary artery bypass grafting; IQR: interquartile range; LIMA: left internal mammary artery; D1: the first diagonal branch; LAD: the left anterior descending artery; RIMA-T: the right internal mammary artery as a t-graft from the left internal mammary artery; M1: the first marginal branch of the circumflex artery; MIDCAB: minimally invasive direct coronary artery bypass; RCA: right coronary artery; RCX: circumflex artery.

Table 2. Preoperative EF and mitral valve pathology.

Patient No.	Preop. EF	Mitral Valve Pathology
1	60%	Mixed regurgitation due to atrial remodeling due to - Long persistent atrial fibrillation (Carpentier type I) and - A2 prolapse due to chordal elongation
2	60%	Mixed regurgitation due to - atrial remodeling due to paroxysmal atrial fibrillation (Carpentier type I) and - local A1 prolapse due to chordal elongation
3	50%	Primary regurgitation due to P3 flail due to P3 chordal rupture
4	37%	Secondary regurgitation due to PML restriction due to LV remodeling and ICM
5	40%	Secondary regurgitation due to PML restriction due to LV remodeling and ICM
6	59%	Secondary regurgitation due to atrial remodeling due to long persistent atrial fibrillation (Carpentier type I)
7	30%	Secondary regurgitation due to AML restriction due to LV remodeling and ICM
8	60	Primary regurgitation due to P2 flail due to P2 chordal rupture
9	60	Primary regurgitation due to P2 flail due to P2 chordal rupture
10	60	Primary regurgitation due to Barlow disease with bileaflet billowing and pronounced P2 prolapse due to chordal elongation

Abbreviations: AML: Anterior Mitral Leaflet; EF: left ventricular ejection fraction; A1, A2, P2, P3: anterior and posterior segments of the mitral leaflets; LV: left ventricle; PML: posterior mitral leaflet; ICM: ischemic cardiomyopathy.

3.2. Procedural Data

3.2.1. Coronary Intervention

Nine patients underwent PCI with stent implantation before the surgery. The median time between PCI and MIMVS was 48 (IQR, 8–63) days. One patient who had previously undergone cardiac surgery underwent the current coronary intervention 48 days after the procedure. Overall, the procedural success rate was 100%. The stents used included Coroflex, Coroflex Blue, Coroflex Blue Ultra, Coroflex ISAR (B. Braun Melsungen AG, Melsungen, Germany), and Xience pro (Abbott Vascular, Santa Clara, CA, USA). There were no periprocedural complications. All patients received dual antiplatelet therapy with acetylsalicylic acid and clopidogrel. Table 3 summarizes the details of the coronary interventions performed.

Table 3. Procedural data.

Patient No.	PCI before or after Surgery	Time Span (Days)	Target Vessel	Number of Stents	Stent Type
1	Before	17	LAD Segment 6	1	80% proximal to DES → BMS (coroflex Blue 3.0/14 proximal to DES)
2	Before	8	RCA Segment 3	1	BMS (Coroflex Blue Ultra 2.5/14)
3	Before	21	D1 Segment 9	1	DES Coroflex ISAER 2.5/14
4	Before	63	RCA multiple segments	2	Segment 1: POBA 4.0 Balloon 10 bar due to previous stent stenosis Segment 2: DES Coroflex ISAR 4.0/15 Segment 3 DES Coroflex ISAR 2.75/19

Table 3. Cont.

Patient No.	PCI before or after Surgery	Time Span (Days)	Target Vessel	Number of Stents	Stent Type
5	Before	66	RCX segment 12	1	DES (Xience pro 2.75/12)
6	Before	62	RCX segment 13	1	DES (Coroflex ISAR 3.0/19)
7	Before	61	LAD segment 6	1	DES (Coroflex ISAR 3.0/14)
9	After	48	RCA segment 2	1	BMS (Coroflex Blue 4.0/25)
10	Before	7	RCX segment 13	2	2x BMS (2x Coroflex 2.5/9)
11	Before	3	LAD segment 7	1	BMS (Coroflex 3.0/25)

Abbreviations: PCI: percutaneous coronary angioplasty; LAD: left anterior descending artery; RCA: right coronary artery; D1: the first diagonal branch of LAD; RCX: circumflex artery; DES: drug eluting stent; BMS: bare metal stent; POBA: plain old balloon angioplasty.

3.2.2. Surgical Procedure

MIMVS was performed as previously described [4]. In brief, the patient was brought to the operation theatre, placed under general anesthesia, and intubated with a single-lumen endotracheal tube. The patient was then put on cardiopulmonary bypass (CPB) via femoral arterial and venous cannulae. In case of concomitant tricuspid valve surgery, a second venous cannula was inserted into the right jugular vein. After dissecting pleural adhesions, if present, via an anterolateral minithoracotomy, the CPB was initiated and the heart and aorta were exposed. In eight patients, the aorta was cross-clamped with a Valve Gate™ transthoracic aortic clamp (Geister, Tuttlingen, Germany) and antegrade Bretschneider's Custodiol® crystalloid cardioplegia (Dr. Franz Köhler Chemie, Bensheim, Germany) was administered via the aortic root, followed by left atriotomy and exposure of the mitral valve with a Valve Gate™ special minimally invasive atrial retractor (Geister, Tuttlingen, Germany). In one patient with extensive intrapericardial adhesions and in one of two patients who had previously undergone coronary surgery, cross-clamping of the aorta was not possible due to excessive adhesions; therefore, atriotomy and mitral valve exposure were performed in a beating heart. In these two patients, the heart was put into ventricular fibrillation directly before introducing the mitral ring into the left atrium to prevent an air embolism after achieving a competent valve. After completion of the mitral valve repair, the left atrium was closed and the aortic clamp was removed (or the heart defibrillated in the two aforementioned cases). This was followed by gradual weaning from the cardiopulmonary bypass and wound closure after echocardiographic confirmation of successful valve repair. Table 4 summarizes the surgical details of all the patients.

Table 4. Surgical data.

Patient No	Redo Surgery	Beating Heart Surgery	Surgery on DAPT	Surgery	Repair Technique
1	No	No	No	MV repair	32 mm Ring, A2–A3 plication
2	No	No	Yes	MV repair, Cryoablation	32 mm Ring, A1–P1 edge-to-edge stitch, P1–P2 indentation closure
3	No	No	Yes	MV repair, Cryoablation	32 mm Ring, P2 triangular resection
4	Yes	Yes	Yes	MV repair	36 mm Ring
5	No	Yes	Yes	MV repair	30 mm Ring
6	No	No	Yes	MV and TV repair, Cryoablation	28 mm Ring, 34 mm tricuspid band
7	No	No	Yes	MV repair	32 mm Ring

Table 4. Cont.

Patient No	Redo Surgery	Beating Heart Surgery	Surgery on DAPT	Surgery	Repair Technique
9	Yes	No	No	MV repair	30 mm Ring, P2 triangular resection
10	No	No	Yes	MV repair, PFO–closure	34 mm Ring, P2 triangular resection
11	No	No	Yes	MV repair	32 mm Ring, P2 triangular resection

Abbreviations: DAPT: double antiplatelet therapy; MV: mitral valve; TV: tricuspid valve; PFO: patent foramen ovale.

The median operative time was 230 (IQR, 200–255) minutes. The median CPB time was 144 (IQR, 124–152) minutes. The median ischemic time in patients who underwent aortic cross-clamping was 80 (IQR, 66–89) minutes. All valves were successfully repaired. There were no cases of valve replacement. There was no conversion to sternotomy and no intraoperative complications.

3.3. Postoperative Data Analysis

Table 5 summarizes the postoperative results. There was no case of postoperative low cardiac output requiring inotropic support or mechanical support or of myocardial infarction or postoperative stroke. Two patients developed postoperative delirium. One patient underwent re-thoracotomy for bleeding. Blood transfusion was needed in one patient perioperatively and in five patients during the postoperative period. One of the three patients who underwent ablation regained sinus rhythm, while the other two demonstrated persistent atrial fibrillation. No cases required permanent pacemaker implantation. One patient with postoperative sepsis was successfully treated with antibiotics with no further complications. The median ventilation time was 20 (IQR, 14–24) hours. The median duration of stay in intensive care was 3 (IQR, 2–4) days and the median duration of hospital stay was 8 (IQR, 8–11) days. There was no case of in-hospital mortality. The 30-day survival rate was 100%.

Table 5. Postoperative results.

Variable	Result
Postoperative myocardial infarction	0
Postoperative stroke	0
Postoperative delirium, n	2
Drain volume, mL (IQR)	1100 (850–1450)
Re-thoracotomy for bleeding, n	1
Perioperative blood transfusion, n	1
Postoperative blood transfusion, n	5
Ventilation time, hours (IQR)	10 (14–24)
ICU time, days (IQR)	3 (2–4)
Hospital stay, days (IQR)	8 (8–11)
30-day survival rate, %	100

Abbreviations: IQR: interquartile range.

4. Discussion

Prospective randomized trials did not demonstrate a survival benefit of MIMVS over traditional surgery via sternotomy [1,2,5]. However, previous studies did report better cosmetic results and shorter hospital stays with MIMVS over traditional surgery via sternotomy [1,2]. As both factors are welcomed by both patients and clinicians, an increasing number of patients with mitral valve pathologies are undergoing the procedure via the minimally invasive approach [6–9]; over 50% of those who undergo isolated mitral valve surgery in Germany do so via the minimally invasive approach [9].

Although the recent guidelines on valvular heart disease recommend the CABG procedure in the presence of coronary heart disease (CHD) in patients with primary indications for aortic or mitral valve surgery, they recommend PCI in patients who undergo catheter-based intervention of either valve [3,10]. These recommendations are understandable because the CABG procedure is favorable in patients who undergo sternotomy for the valve surgery and PCI is favorable in those who receive treatment percutaneously. Although previous reports have been published reporting favorable results of a hybrid concept consisting of PCI and MIMVS in different patient cohorts with mitral valve and coronary disease [11–14], there are no recommendations regarding the revascularization strategy in patients who might undergo MIMVS in the presence of adequate expertise.

In this study, we evaluated the decision-making process and results of this hybrid concept. The strategy of the heart team was to analyze CHD independent from the mitral valve pathology. If CHD was to be treated endovascularly according to the recent guidelines with no mitral valve pathology, this hybrid concept was suggested [3]. The rationale behind this concept was to not deny the patient mitral valve repair via a favorable approach due to coronary pathology that would have been otherwise treated endovascularly with expected good results. Additionally, the rationale is also to facilitate the approach to the mitral valve in re-do procedures after a previous CABG with patent grafts where avoiding re-sternotomy is of special benefit to avoid graft injury. The results of this study demonstrate that this concept is a viable option in the presence of adequate expertise in MIMVS. Based on this study, we developed a simple decision-making flowchart to help in patient selection (Figure 1).

Another important aspect is the sequence of the procedures. On one hand, it might be surgically favorable to perform the surgical procedure before initiating double antiplatelet therapy (DPAT) after endovascular therapy for CHD because randomized controlled trials and retrospective studies have demonstrated higher rates of postoperative bleeding in patients on DPAT [15–19]. On the other hand, it is crucial to ensure adequate coronary perfusion before the surgery or at least ensure adequate myocardial protection with cardioplegia and avoid periprocedural myocardial infarction because previous publications have demonstrated a higher rate of perioperative myocardial infarctions in patients whose diseased coronary vessels were not addressed [20,21]. In our study cohort, we generally opted to perform PCI first to also confirm the success of myocardial revascularization before MIMVS.

Regarding the optimum timeframe between PCI and MIMVS, the heart team unfortunately did not reach a consensus at the time of performing the procedures. Post-PCI clopidogrel therapy was stopped 5 days before the surgery in patients who were operated on after more than 30 days of PCI according to the ESC/EACTS guidelines [22]. In patients with severe valvular symptoms who were operated on within 1 month of PCI, surgery was performed under DAPT. Our analysis did not demonstrate higher bleeding tendency in these patients. Furthermore, the analysis did not reveal periprocedural myocardial infarctions or low cardiac output syndrome, which reflect adequate myocardial perfusion and protection. Therefore, we believe that it is advisable to first address the CHD to ensure successful revascularization before surgery and to optimize myocardial protection during surgery.

The patients who had previously undergone CABG and were to undergo re-do surgery represented a special cohort. In the first patient, the heart team preferred to perform the mitral valve surgery first to avoid the bleeding tendencies in re-do situations. As the surgical team did not face increased bleeding tendency in this patient, the second patient underwent PCI first and then surgery, which was performed without complications. In hindsight, while believing that PCI should precede MIMVS, we also believe that it is advisable to plan PCI well before MIMVS to be able to safely stop DAPT before the surgery to decrease the bleeding risk without highly increasing the risk of stent thrombosis.

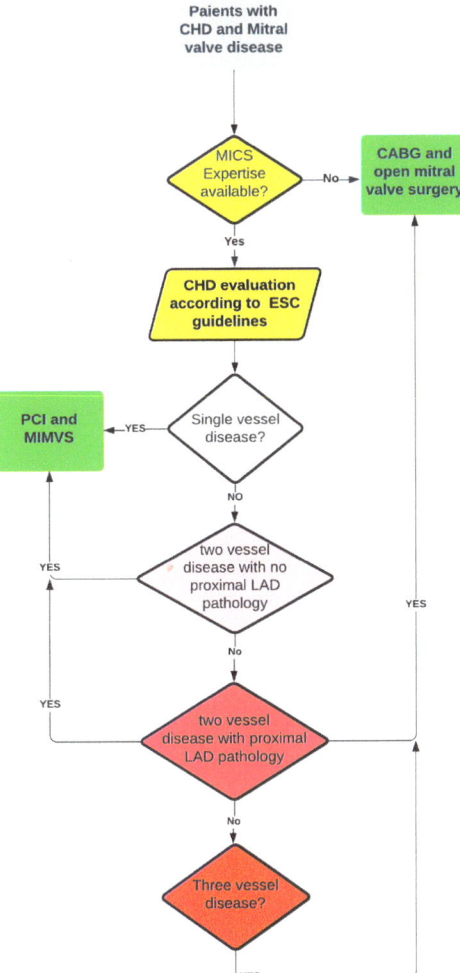

Figure 1. Decision-making flowchart for patient selection. Abbreviations: CHD: coronary heart disease; MICS: minimally invasive cardiac surgery; CABG: coronary artery bypass grafting; ESC: European Society of Cardiology; LAD: left anterior descending artery; PCI: percutaneous coronary intervention; MIMVS: minimally invasive mitral valve surgery.

This study has several limitations. It was a single center study that included a small number of patients, and procedures were not randomly assigned. To our knowledge, there are no previous studies that have evaluated the feasibility of hybrid PCI and MIMVS in similar cohorts. Therefore, further studies with larger patient numbers are required to corroborate the results of the present study and to draw more robust conclusions. Furthermore, the patient management protocol did not adhere to a standardized protocol regarding the timeframe between the procedures. Further studies should adhere to a standardized timeframe to provide clearer recommendations. Nevertheless, MIMVS might be more tolerant of DAPT with less restrictive indications for surgery under DAPT. This is yet to be confirmed in further studies.

5. Conclusions

A hybrid concept of PCI and MIMVS is feasible in patients with mitral valve pathology and single vessel coronary disease and can be considered if the team members have sufficient expertise in MIMVS. Future studies should also evaluate whether this recommendation is feasible for patients with multivessel disease, so that for patients with combined mitral valve and coronary pathologies, with the availability of adequate expertise in MIMVS, the choice of revascularization strategy can be evaluated independent from the mitral valve pathology.

Based on the results of this report, in centers with expertise in MIMVS, the coronary pathology and the choice revascularization strategy should be made independent from the mitral valve pathology. In patients whose coronary pathology is suitable for PCI, a hybrid PCI and MIMVS should be considered.

Author Contributions: Conceptualization, A.J.R. and H.N.; methodology, A.J.R., H.N. and M.M.-L.; software, T.G.; validation, M.M.-L.; formal analysis, T.G.; investigation, T.G.; data curation, T.G.; writing—original draft preparation, M.V.; writing—review and editing, M.I. and T.G.; supervision, A.J.R. All authors have read and agreed to the published version of the manuscript.

Funding: This research received no external funding.

Institutional Review Board Statement: The study was conducted in accordance with the Declaration of Helsinki and approved by the Institutional Review Board (or Ethics Committee) of Landesärztekammer Hessen (protocol code 2023-3337-evBO; date of approval 21.06.2023).

Informed Consent Statement: Patient consent was waived due to the retrospective nature of the study with data analysis confined to the intrahospital data.

Data Availability Statement: The data presented in this study are available on request from the corresponding author. The data are not publicly available due to data privacy regulation of the ethical committee.

Conflicts of Interest: The authors declare no conflict of interest.

References

1. Speziale, G.; Nasso, G.; Esposito, G.; Conte, M.; Greco, E.; Fattouch, K.; Fiore, F.; Del Giglio, M.; Coppola, R.; Tavazzi, L. Results of mitral valve repair for Barlow disease (bileaflet prolapse) via right minithoracotomy versus conventional median sternotomy: A randomized trial. *J. Thorac. Cardiovasc Surg.* **2011**, *142*, 77–83. [CrossRef]
2. Dogan, S.; Aybek, T.; Risteski, P.S.; Detho, F.; Rapp, A.; Wimmer-Greinecker, G.; Moritz, A. Minimally invasive port access versus conventional mitral valve surgery: Prospective randomized study. *Ann. Thorac. Surg.* **2005**, *79*, 492–498. [CrossRef] [PubMed]
3. Sousa-Uva, M.; Neumann, F.J.; Ahlsson, A.; Alfonso, F.; Banning, A.P.; Benedetto, U.; Byrne, R.A.; Collet, J.P.; Falk, V.; Head, S.J.; et al. 2018 ESC/EACTS Guidelines on myocardial revascularization. *Eur. J. Cardio-Thoracic Surg.* **2019**, *55*, 4–90. [CrossRef] [PubMed]
4. Chitwood, R.W.; Rodriguez, E. Minimally invasive and robotic mitral valve surgery. In *Cardiac Sugery in the Adult*, 3rd ed.; Cohen, L.H., Ed.; McGraw-Hill: New York, NY, USA, 2008; pp. 1079–1100.
5. Nasso, G.; Bonifazi, R.; Romano, V.; Bartolomucci, F.; Rosano, G.; Massari, F.; Fattouch, K.; Del Prete, G.; Riccioni, G.; Del Giglio, M.; et al. Three-year results of repaired Barlow mitral valves via right minithoracotomy versus median sternotomy in a randomized trial. *Cardiology* **2014**, *128*, 97–105. [CrossRef] [PubMed]
6. Beckmann, A.; Funkat, A.K.; Lewandowski, J.; Frie, M.; Ernst, M.; Hekmat, K.; Schiller, W.; Gummert, J.; Welz, A. German Heart Surgery Report 2015: The Annual Updated Registry of the German Society for Thoracic and Cardiovascular Surgery. *Thorac. Cardiovasc Surg.* **2016**, *64*, 462–474. [PubMed]
7. Beckmann, A.; Funkat, A.K.; Lewandowski, J.; Frie, M.; Ernst, M.; Hekmat, K.; Schiller, W.; Gummert, J.; Harringer, W. German heart surgery report 2016: The annual updated registry of the German society, for thoracic and cardiovascular surgery. *Thorac. Cardiovasc Surg.* **2017**, *65*, 505–518. [PubMed]
8. Beckmann, A.; Meyer, R.; Lewandowski, J.; Frie, M.; Markewitz, A.; Harringer, W. German heart surgery report 2017: The annual updated registry of the German society for thoracic and cardiovascular surgery. *Thorac. Cardiovasc Surg.* **2018**, *66*, 608–621. [PubMed]
9. Beckmann, A.; Meyer, R.; Lewandowski, J.; Markewitz, A.; Harringer, W. German heart surgery report 2018: The annual updated registry of the German society for thoracic and cardiovascular surgery. *Thorac. Cardiovasc Surgeon.* **2019**, *67*, 331–344. [CrossRef]

10. Baumgartner, H.; Falk, V.; Bax, J.J.; De Bonis, M.; Hamm, C.; Holm, P.J.; Iung, B.; Lancellotti, P.; Lansac, E.; Rodriguez Muñoz, D.; et al. 2017 ESC/EACTS Guidelines for the management of valvular heart disease. *Eur. Heart J.* **2017**, *38*, 2739–2786. [CrossRef]
11. Santana, O.; Xydas, S.; Williams, R.F.; Mawad, M.; Heimowitz, T.B.; Pineda, A.M.; Goldman, H.S.; Mihos, C.G. Hybrid approach of percutaneous coronary intervention followed by minimally invasive mitral valve surgery: A 5-year single-center experience. *J. Thorac. Dis.* **2017**, *9*, 595–601. [CrossRef]
12. Santana, O.; Pineda, A.M.; Cortes-Bergoderi, M.; Mihos, C.G.; Beohar, N.; Lamas, G.A.; Lamelas, J. Hybrid approach of percutaneous coronary intervention followed by minimally invasive valve operations. *Ann. Thorac. Surg.* **2014**, *97*, 2049–2055. [CrossRef] [PubMed]
13. Leacche, M.; Umakanthan, R.; Zhao, D.X.; Byrne, J.G. Surgical update hybrid procedures, do they have a role? *Circ. Cardiovasc Interv.* **2010**, *3*, 511–518. [CrossRef] [PubMed]
14. Mihos, C.G.; Santana, O.; Pineda, A.M.; Stone, G.W.; Hasty, F.; Beohar, N. Percutaneous coronary intervention followed by minimally invasive mitral valve surgery in ischemic mitral regurgitation. *Innov. Technol. Tech. Cardio-Thorac. Vasc. Surg.* **2015**, *10*, 394–397.
15. Tomšič, A.; Schotborgh, M.A.; Manshanden, J.S.J.; Li, W.W.L.; de Mol, B.A.J.M. Coronary artery bypass grafting-related bleeding complications in patients treated with dual antiplatelet treatment. *Eur. J. CardioThorac. Surg.* **2016**, *50*, 849–856. [CrossRef] [PubMed]
16. Hansson, E.C.; Jidéus, L.; Åberg, B.; Bjursten, H.; Dreifaldt, M.; Holmgren, A.; Ivert, T.; Nozohoor, S.; Barbu, M.; Svedjeholm, R.; et al. Coronary artery bypass grafting-related bleeding complications in patients treated with ticagrelor or clopidogrel: A nationwide study. *Eur. Heart J.* **2016**, *37*, 189–197. [CrossRef] [PubMed]
17. Smith, P.K.; Goodnough, L.T.; Levy, J.H.; Poston, R.S.; Short, M.A.; Weerakkody, G.J.; Lenarz, L.A. Mortality benefit with prasugrel in the TRITON-TIMI 38 coronary artery bypass grafting cohort: Risk-adjusted retrospective data analysis. *J. Am. Coll. Cardiol.* **2012**, *60*, 388–396. [CrossRef] [PubMed]
18. Held, C.; Åsenblad, N.; Bassand, J.P.; Becker, R.C.; Cannon, C.P.; Claeys, M.J.; Harrington, R.A.; Horrow, J.; Husted, S.; James, S.K.; et al. Ticagrelor versus clopidogrel in patients with acute coronary syndromes undergoing coronary artery bypass surgery results from the PLATO (Platelet Inhibition and Patient Outcomes) trial. *J. Am. Coll. Cardiol.* **2011**, *57*, 672–684. [CrossRef] [PubMed]
19. Fox, K.A.A.; Mehta, S.R.; Peters, R.; Zhao, F.; Lakkis, N.; Gersh, B.J.; Yusuf, S. 'Benefits and risks of the combination of clopidogrel and aspirin in patients undergoing surgical revascularization for non-ST-elevation acute coronary syndrome: The Clopidogrel in Unstable angina to prevent Recurrent ischemic Events (CURE) Trial. *Circulation* **2004**, *110*, 1202–1208. [CrossRef]
20. Alamanni, F.; Dainese, L.; Naliato, M.; Gregu, S.; Agrifoglio, M.; Polvani, G.L.; Biglioli, P.; Parolari, A.; Monzino OPCAB Investigators. On- and off-pump coronary surgery and perioperative myocardial infarction: An issue between incomplete and extensive revascularization. *Eur. J. Cardio-Thorac. Surg.* **2008**, *34*, 118–126. [CrossRef]
21. Leviner, D.B.; Torregrossa, G.; Puskas, J.D. Incomplete revascularization: What the surgeon needs to know. *Ann. Cardio-Thorac. Surg.* **2018**, *7*, 463–469.
22. Valgimigli, M.; Bueno, H.; Byrne, R.A.; Collet, J.P.; Costa, F.; Jeppsson, A.; Jüni, P.; Kastrati, A.; Kolh, P.; Mauri, L.; et al. 2017 ESC focused update on dual antiplatelet therapy in coronary artery disease developed in collaboration with EACTS. *Eur. J. Cardio-Thorac. Surg.* **2018**, *53*, 34–78. [CrossRef]

Disclaimer/Publisher's Note: The statements, opinions and data contained in all publications are solely those of the individual author(s) and contributor(s) and not of MDPI and/or the editor(s). MDPI and/or the editor(s) disclaim responsibility for any injury to people or property resulting from any ideas, methods, instructions or products referred to in the content.

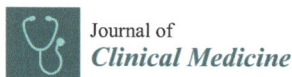 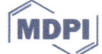

Article

Minimally Invasive Isolated Aortic Valve Replacement in a Potential TAVI Cohort of Patients Aged ≥ 75 Years: A Propensity-Matched Analysis

Ali Taghizadeh-Waghefi [1,2,*], Asen Petrov [1,2], Philipp Jatzke [3], Manuel Wilbring [1,2], Utz Kappert [1,2], Klaus Matschke [1,2], Konstantin Alexiou [1,2,†] and Sebastian Arzt [1,2,†]

1. Medical Faculty "Carl Gustav Carus", Technical University of Dresden, 01307 Dresden, Germany
2. Center of Minimally Invasive Cardiac Surgery, University Heart Center Dresden, Faculty of Medicine, Technical University of Dresden, 01037 Dresden, Germany
3. Anesthesiology and Intensive Care Medicine, Dresden University Hospital, Faculty of Medicine, Technical University of Dresden, 01307 Dresden, Germany
* Correspondence: swaghefi@gmail.com
† These authors contributed equally to this work.

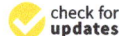

Citation: Taghizadeh-Waghefi, A.; Petrov, A.; Jatzke, P.; Wilbring, M.; Kappert, U.; Matschke, K.; Alexiou, K.; Arzt, S. Minimally Invasive Isolated Aortic Valve Replacement in a Potential TAVI Cohort of Patients Aged ≥ 75 Years: A Propensity-Matched Analysis. *J. Clin. Med.* **2023**, *12*, 4963. https://doi.org/10.3390/jcm12154963

Academic Editors: Maurizio Taramasso, Antonio Miceli and Omer Dzemali

Received: 26 February 2023
Revised: 9 July 2023
Accepted: 17 July 2023
Published: 28 July 2023

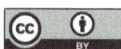

Copyright: © 2023 by the authors. Licensee MDPI, Basel, Switzerland. This article is an open access article distributed under the terms and conditions of the Creative Commons Attribution (CC BY) license (https://creativecommons.org/licenses/by/4.0/).

Abstract: (1) Background and Objectives: Transcatheter aortic valve implantation is guideline-recommended from the age of 75. However, this European guideline recommendation is based on limited evidence, since no interaction between age and primary outcome has been found in guideline-stated references. This study aimed to compare the short-term outcomes of minimally invasive isolated aortic valve replacement in patients aged ≥ 75 with those of younger patients; (2) Patients and Methods: This retrospective cohort study included 1339 patients who underwent minimally invasive isolated aortic valve replacement at our facility between 2014 and 2022. This cohort was divided into two age-based groups: <75 and ≥75 years. Operative morbidity and mortality were compared between groups. Further analysis was performed using propensity score matching; (3) Results: After matching, 347 pairs of patients were included and analyzed. Despite the higher EuroSCORE II in the ≥75 group (2.2 ± 1.3% vs. 1.80 ± 1.34%, $p \leq 0.001$), the 30-day mortality (1.4% vs. 1.2%; $p = 0.90$) and major adverse cardiac and cerebrovascular events, such as perioperative myocardial infarction (0.0% vs. 1.2%, $p = 0.12$) and stroke (1.4% vs. 2.6%, $p = 0.06$), were comparable between both treatment groups; (4) Conclusions: Minimally invasive aortic valve replacement is a safe treatment method for patients aged ≥ 75. Our results indicate that the unilateral cut-off of 75 years is not a limiting factor for performing minimally invasive aortic valve replacement.

Keywords: surgical aortic valve replacement; minimally invasive aortic valve replacement; minimally invasive surgery; outcomes; TAVI

1. Introduction

The 2021 European Society of Cardiology and European Association for Cardio-Thoracic Surgery guidelines for the treatment of valvular heart disease recommend an age cut-off of ≥75 years as a decision-making criterion for selecting therapeutic procedures for severe aortic stenosis (AS) in favor of transcatheter aortic valve implantation (TAVI) [1]. The Class I recommendation with level of evidence grade A is notable in this regard. Previous clinical studies that form the basis of this recommendation relate to the PARTNER [2–4], SURTAVI [5], Corevalve high-risk trial [6] and NOTION [7] trials. However, except for the NOTION trial, where patients aged ≥ 70 years were randomly assigned to surgical aortic valve replacement (SAVR) or TAVI, these studies did not primarily evaluate age-based outcomes. Therefore, this recommendation on patient age has a high risk of methodological error. Furthermore, an evidence-based answer to whether patients ≥ 75 years derive a clear benefit from the TAVI procedure remains elusive. Not to be neglected are the progressive advances in surgical techniques for isolated aortic valve replacement, which eventually led to the development of minimally invasive aortic valve replacement (MIAVR). MIAVR is increasingly being performed as an alternative to standard sternotomy to meet the rising patient demand for faster postoperative recovery and improved quality of life. Therefore, this study reports the short-term postoperative results and outcomes of MIAVR in patients aged ≥ 75 with a life expectancy of >5 years compared to younger patients.

2. Materials and Methods

2.1. Patient Population, Study Design and Ethics Statement

This study is a retrospective observational cohort analysis of consecutive patients undergoing minimally invasive aortic valve surgery according to the inclusion criteria. Data were collected from the hospital database. This study was reviewed and approved by the local Ethics Board (EK—Nr. 298092012).

Generally, all patients being admitted with a symptomatic high-grade aortic valve stenosis undergo a Heart Team decision process. During this decision-making process, patients who are likely to have a life expectancy of ≤ 5 years due to their age or comorbidities are usually assigned to a TAVI procedure. The remaining patients are primarily screened for MIAVR. This prospective decision making is represented in the retrospectively analyzed cohort, according to the flow chart depicted below (Figure 1). Sternotomy patients were ruled out to exclude any selection bias.

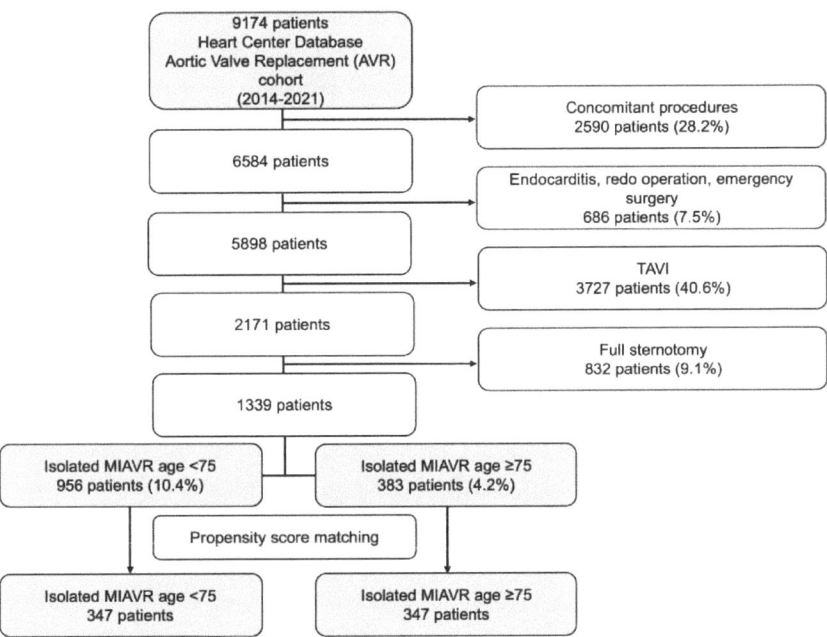

Figure 1. Flow diagram of the study population. Abbreviations: MIAVR, minimally invasive aortic valve replacement.

Between 2014 and 2022, 2171 patients underwent elective isolated primary SAVR at our facility due to degenerative aortic valve disease. Eight hundred thirty-two patients who underwent full sternotomy were excluded. Therefore, this retrospective analysis included 1339 patients who underwent isolated MIAVR. This cohort was divided into two age-based groups: <75 years and ≥ 75 years. Demographic, clinical, surgical and short-term postoperative outcome data were obtained from medical records retrospectively. Figure 1 shows the patient selection process as a flow chart.

2.2. Surgical MIAVR Access Routes

Three different access routes for MIAVR are performed at our facility (Figure 2). The choice of minimally invasive surgical approach was based on the surgeon's preference and the patient's anatomic characteristics, which were assessed using electrocardiogram (ECG)-gated computed tomography angiography of the thorax, abdomen and pelvis. The surgical access routes consisted of upper partial sternotomy (UPS), right anterolateral thoracotomy (RAT) and right lateral thoracotomy (RLA). In UPS, a 5–10 cm median skin incision is made below the sternal notch, followed by a J-shaped division of the upper part of the sternum up to the level of the third or fourth intercostal space. RAT involves a 5 cm skin incision and dissection of the pectoralis and intercostal muscles and the right mammary artery along the second intercostal space. RLA uses a 5 cm skin incision made along the right anterior axillary line, followed by dissection of serratus anterior and intercostal muscle and opening of the third or fourth intercostal space [8]. Regardless of the surgical access route, extra-corporal circulation was established via the femoral vessels, placing antegrade cardioplegia cannula in the ascending aorta and the left ventricular venting line via the right superior pulmonary vein.

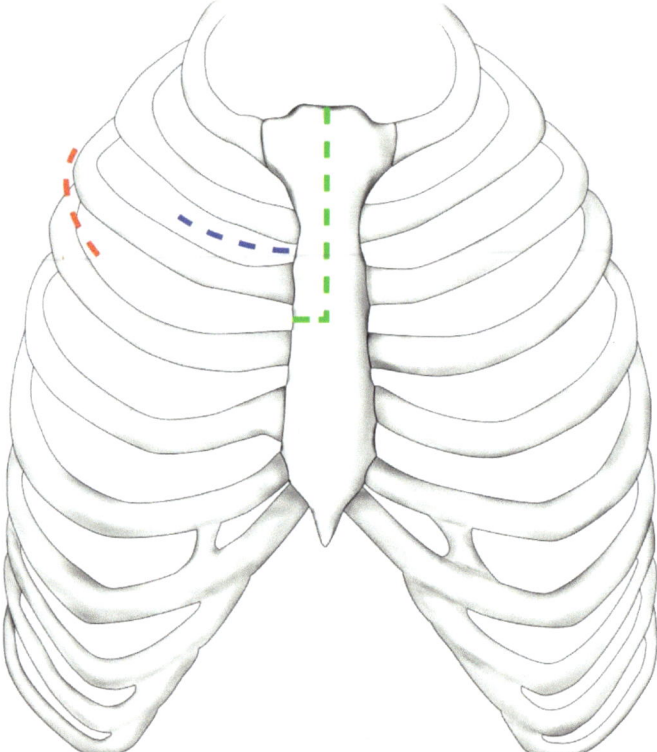

Figure 2. Surgical access routes. Upper partial sternotomy (green dashed line), right anterolateral thoracotomy (blue dashed line), right lateral thoracotomy (red dashed line).

2.3. Statistical Analysis

Continuous data are expressed as mean ± standard deviation (SD). Categorial variables are presented as numbers and percentages. All continuous variable data were checked for normality using the Kolmogorov–Smirnov test with Lilliefors significance correction (type I error = 10%). Normally distributed variables were tested for variance heteroscedasticity using Levene's test (type I error = 5%). Normally distributed variables with homogeneous variance were compared between subgroups using independent two-sample *t*-tests. Normally distributed variables with heterogeneous variance were compared using Welch's *t*-test. Non-normally distributed and ordinal variables were compared using Mann–Whitney's U-test. Dichotomous variables were compared using Fisher's exact test. Other categorical variables were compared using the χ^2 test (either exact or with Monte Carlo simulation). For individual categories, deviations from the expected frequencies are presented as adjusted residuals. Since the type I error was not adjusted for multiple testing, the results of inferential statistics are descriptive only, and the use of the term "significant" in the description of the study results always reflects only a local $p < 0.05$ but no error probability below 5%.

A bias-reduced subset of the full data set was obtained by propensity score matching of the following variables: sex, body mass index (BMI), preoperative left ventricular ejection fraction (LVEF), estimated creatinine clearance according to the Cockcroft–Gault equation (CRCL), preoperative New York Heart Association (NYHA) classification, diabetes mellitus, pulmonary arterial hypertension, coronary artery disease, peripheral occlusive arterial disease and chronic obstructive pulmonary disease (COPD). A maximum allowable difference between two patients of 0.08 was defined to ensure good matches. The choice of the caliper value of 0.08 was based on ensuring that the two groups being compared are as similar as possible while also maximizing the number of matches. It was started with a higher caliper value, which was gradually decreased until the balance between the similarity (no statistically relevant differences between the propensity-score-matching parameters regarding the groups) and the number of matches was satisfactory. Hence, the stated caliper value was used for the matching. The standardized differences are shown in Table 1. Figure 3 shows the covariate balance before and after adjustment. Statistical analyses were performed using the open-source R statistical software (v.4.1.2).

Table 1. Standardized differences of the variables.

	Before Matching	After Matching
BMI (kg/m^2)	0.152	0.055
Preoperative LVEF (%)	0.038	0.039
Estimated creatinine clearance (mL/min)	1.023	0.079
NYHA I	0.046	0.023
NYHA II	0.139	0.048
NYHA III	0.150	0.035
NYHA IV	<0.001	0.029
Sex	0.170	0.075
Diabetes (no/yes)	0.167	0.048
Pulmonary hypertension (no/yes)	0.251	0.061
Coronary artery disease (no/yes)	0.380	0.012
Peripheral vascular disease (no/yes)	0.016	0.032
Chronic obstructive pulmonary disease (no/yes)	0.008	0.020

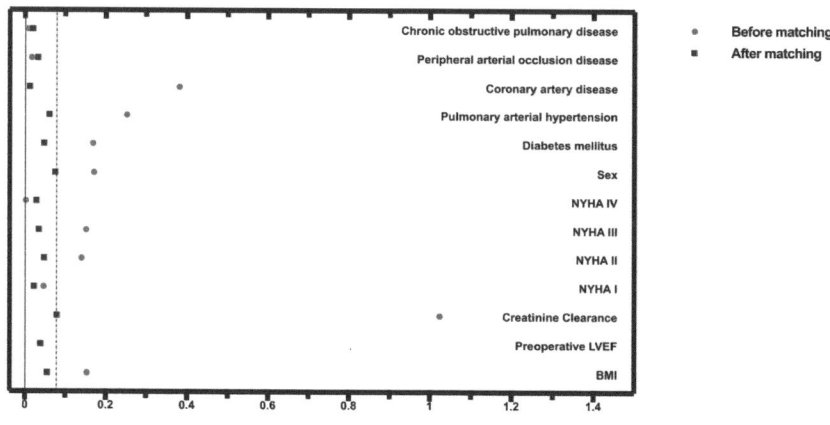

Figure 3. The covariate balance before and after propensity score matching. The dashed line represents the matching caliper of 0.08.

3. Results

3.1. Patient Baseline Characteristics

Between January 2014 and February 2022, 1339 patients underwent MIAVR and were divided into two age-based groups based on a cut-off of 75 years, with 956 patients in the isolated MIAVR < 75 group (mean age = 64.2 ± 8.1) and 383 patients in the isolated MIAVR ≥ 75 group (mean age = 77.3 ± 1.7). The sex distribution differed in the two groups, with more males in the <75 group (65.2%) than in the ≥75 group (56.9%; $p \leq 0.01$). Patients in the ≥75 group had a significantly higher mean calculated risk stratification score for mortality (EuroSCORE II = 2.25 ± 1.31% and STS-PROM score = 1.91 ± 0.9%) than those in the <75 group (1.38 ± 1.03 with $p \leq 0.001$ and 1.14 ± 0.67 with $p \leq 0.001$, respectively). They were also more likely to be NYHA class III or IV and to have more comorbidities, such as arterial hypertension, diabetes mellitus, coronary artery disease, pulmonary arterial hypertension, renal insufficiency, significant carotid artery stenosis (stenosis ≥ 50% measured according to the NASCET criteria) and atrial fibrillation. There were significantly more smokers in the <75 group than in the ≥75 group.

We could propensity score match 347 patients from each group in the full cohort according to the above-mentioned variables, so that both groups had similar baseline characteristics. After the matching procedure, the main significant differences between the <75 and ≥75 groups were age (77.2 ± 1.7 vs. 67.8 ± 5.9; $p \leq 0.001$), as expected, and under the influence of age, the calculated risk stratification scores for mortality (EuroSCORE II 2.2 ± 1.3% vs. 1.80 ± 1.34%, $p \leq 0.001$; STS-PROM score 1.9 ± 0.9% vs. 1.5 ± 0.8%, $p \leq 0.001$). Moreover, patients in the ≥75 group more frequently had arterial hypertension, significant carotid stenosis and implanted permanent pacemakers than patients in the <75 group. Patients with preoperative terminal-dialysis-dependent renal insufficiency were significantly more common in the <75 group than in the ≥75 group. Other baseline characteristics did not differ significantly after matching. The baseline characteristics of the pre-matched and propensity-matched groups are shown in Table 2.

Table 2. Baseline characteristics.

	Pre-Matched Cohort			Propensity-Score-Matched Cohort		
	Isolated MIAVR <75 (n = 956)	Isolated MIAVR ≥75 (n = 383)	p	Isolated MIAVR <75 (n = 347)	Isolated MIAVR ≥75 (n = 347)	p
Age (years), mean ± SD	64.2 ± 8.1	77.3 ± 1.7	*≤0.001* **	67.8 ± 5.9	77.2 ± 1.7	*<0.001* **
Sex (male), n (%)	623 (65.2)	218 (56.9)	*≤0.01* *	186 (53.6)	199 (57.3)	0.36
Height (cm), mean ± SD	171.2 ± 9.3	168.8 ± 9.3	*≤0.001* **	167.5 ± 9.0	168.7 ± 9.4	0.09
Weight (kg), mean ± SD	83.9 ± 16.7	79.5 ± 13.8	*≤0.001* **	79.4 ± 15.4	79.9 ± 13.9	0.24
BMI (kg/m^2), mean ± SD	28.6 ± 5.1	27.9 ± 4.2	0.10	28.3 ± 4.9	28.0 ± 4.2	≥0.99
Arterial hypertension, n (%)	866 (90.6)	378 (98.7)	*≤0.001* **	332 (95.7)	343 (98.8)	*0.02* *
Diabetes mellitus, n (%)	263 (27.5)	135 (35.2)	*0.02* *	119 (34.3)	127 (36.6)	0.91
Dyslipidemia, n (%)	565 (59.1)	245 (64.0)	0.11	212 (61.1)	228 (65.7)	0.24
Coronary artery disease, n (%)	210 (22.0)	150 (39.2)	*≤0.001* **	132 (38.0)	130 (37.5)	0.77
LVEF (%), mean ± SD	57.3 ± 11.1	57 ± 9.6	0.79	58.1 ± 11.1	57.7 ± 9.6	0.39
COPD, n (%)	82 (8.6)	32 (8.4)	≥0.99	33 (9.5)	31 (8.9)	0.90
Pulmonary arterial hypertension, n (%)	100 (10.5)	74 (19.3)	*≤0.001* **	55 (15.9)	63 (18.2)	0.45
Renal insufficiency, n (%)	118 (12.3)	107 (27.9)	*≤0.001* **	97 (28.0)	83 (23.9)	0.26
Hemodialysis, n (%)	10 (1.0)	0 (0.0)	0.07	7 (2.0)	0 (0.0)	*0.02* *
CRCL (mL/min), mean ± SD	91.4 ± 28.0	66.9 ± 19.0	*≤0.001* **	70.5 ± 19.5	68.7 ± 18.8	0.06
PAOD, n (%)	37 (3.9)	16 (4.2)	0.54	11 (3.2)	13 (3.7)	0.84
Carotid artery stenosis > 50%, n (%)	25 (2.6)	34 (8.9)	*≤0.001* **	132 (38)	130 (37.5)	*0.02* *
TIA, n (%)	22 (2.3)	9 (2.3)	≥0.99	10 (2.9)	9 (2.6)	≥0.99
Ischemic stroke, n (%)	39 (4.0)	23 (6.0)	0.14	15 (4.3)	22 (6.4)	0.25
Atrial fibrillation, n (%)	94 (9.8)	79 (20.7)	*≤0.001* **	47 (13.5)	26 (6.1)	0.22
Pacemaker, n (%)	22 (2.3)	21 (5.5)	*≤0.01* *	7 (2.0)	21 (6.1)	*0.01* *
Smoker status, n (%)	149 (15.6)	29 (7.6)	*≤0.001* **	37 (10.7)	26 (7.5)	0.19
NYHA class III or IV, n (%)	531 (55.5)	241 (62.9)	*≤0.01* *	211 (60.8)	218 (62.8)	0.59
EuroSCORE II (%), mean ± SD	1.38 ± 1.0	2.25 ± 1.3	*≤0.001* **	1.8 ± 1.3	2.2 ± 1.3	*≤0.001* **
STS-PROM Score, mean ± SD	1.1 ± 0.7	1.9 ± 0.9	*≤0.001* **	1.5 ± 0.8	1.9 ± 0.9	*≤0.001* **

Note: Bold and italic values indicate statistical significance: *, $p \leq 0.05$; **, $p \leq 0.01$. Abbreviations: MIAVR, minimally invasive aortic valve replacement; SD, standard deviation; BMI, body mass index; LVEF, left ventricular ejection fraction; COPD, chronic obstructive pulmonary disease; CRCL, calculated creatinine clearance according to the Cockcroft-Gault equation; PAOD, peripheral arterial occlusion disease; TIA, transient ischemic attack; NYHA, New York Heart Association; STS-PROM, Society of Thoracic Surgeons predicted risk of mortality.

3.2. Unadjusted Outcomes

Significantly more patients underwent MIAVR through the RAT surgical access route in the ≥75 group (42.0%) than in the <75 group (34.6%; $p \leq 0.05$; Figure 4). There were no significant differences in the use of the other two surgical access routes between groups. As expected, mechanical valve prostheses were implanted more frequently in the <75 group than in the ≥75 group ($p \leq 0.05$). However, significantly more rapid deployment bioprosthetic valves (RDV) were implanted in the ≥75 group than in the <75 group ($p \leq 0.05$; Figure 5). Among the procedural data, there was a significantly longer cardiopulmonary bypass time (CPBT; 66.9 ± 21.8 vs. 64.4 ± 24.5; $p = 0.02$) and aortic cross-clamp time (ACCT; 46.8 ± 16.5 vs. 43.6 ± 14.8; $p \leq 0.001$) in the <75 group than in the ≥75 group (Figure 6). The procedural and intraoperative data are summarized in Tables 3 and 4.

Table 3. Procedural and intraoperative data.

	Pre-Matched Cohort			Propensity-Score-Matched Cohort		
	Isolated MIAVR < 75 (n = 956)	Isolated MIAVR ≥ 75 (n = 383)	p	Isolated MIAVR < 75 (n = 347)	Isolated MIAVR ≥ 75 (n = 347)	p
Surgical access route [†]						
- UPS, n (%)	307 (32.1)	114 (29.8)		110 (31.7)	107 (30.8)	
- RAT, n (%)	331 (34.6)	161 (42.0)	*0.03* *	117 (33.7)	142 (40.9)	0.10
- RLA, n (%)	318 (33.3)	108 (28.2)		120 (34.6)	98 (28.2)	
Prosthesis size (mm), mean ± SD	23.9 ± 2.0	23.8 ± 2.0	0.35	186 (53.6)	199 (57.3)	0.36
STST (min), mean ± SD	171.2 ± 9.3	79.5 ± 13.9	0.44	167.5 ± 9.0	168.7 ± 9.4	0.09
CPBT (min), mean ± SD	66.9 ± 21.8	64.4 ± 24.5	*0.02* *	79.4 ± 15.4	79.9 ± 13.9	0.24
ACCT (min), mean ± SD	46.8 ± 16.5	43.6 ± 14.8	*≤0.001* **	28.3 ± 4.9	28.0 ± 4.2	≥0.99
Prosthesis type [†]						
- Mechanical, n (%)	105 (11.0)	1 (0.3)		18 (5.2)	1 (0.3)	
- Bioprosthetic, n (%)	367 (38.4)	144 (37.6)	*≤0.001* **	131 (37.8)	131 (37.8)	*≤0.001* **
- RDV, n (%)	483 (50.6)	238 (62.1)		198 (57.1)	215 (62.0)	

Note: Bold and italic values indicate statistical significance: *, $p \leq 0.05$; **, $p \leq 0.01$; [†], see Table 3 for adjusted residuals. As a consequence of the process of mathematical rounding, wherein percentages are rounded up or down to the nearest tenth decimal place, minute deviations of up to 0.1% from the absolute value of 100% can potentially manifest. Abbreviations: MIAVR, minimally invasive aortic valve replacement; UPS, upper partial sternotomy; RAT, right anterolateral thoracotomy; RLA, right lateral thoracotomy; SD, standard deviation; STST, skin-to-skin time; CPBT, cardiopulmonary bypass time; ACCT, aortic cross-clamp time; RDV, rapid deployment bioprosthetic valve.

Table 4. Surgical access route and prosthesis type (adjusted residuals for deviations from expected frequencies).

	Pre-Matched Cohort			Propensity-Score-Matched Cohort		
	Isolated MIAVR < 75 (n = 956)	Isolated MIAVR ≥ 75 (n = 383)	p	Isolated MIAVR < 75 (n = 347)	Isolated MIAVR ≥ 75 (n = 347)	p
Surgical access route						
- UPS, asr	0.8	−0.8	>0.05	-	-	>0.05
- RAT, asr	**−2.5**	**2.5**	**≤0.05**	-	-	>0.05
- RLA, asr	1.8	108 (28.2)	>0.05	-	-	>0.05
Prosthesis type						
- Mechanical, asr	**6.6**	**−6.6**	**≤0.05**	**4.0**	**−4.0**	**≤0.05**
- Bioprosthetic, asr	0.3	−0.3	>0.05	0	0	>0.05
- RDV, n (%), asr	**−3.8**	**3.8**	**≤0.05**	−1.3	1.3	>0.05

Note: Bold values indicate statistical significance. Abbreviation: MIAVR, minimally invasive aortic valve replacement; asr, adjusted standardized residuals.

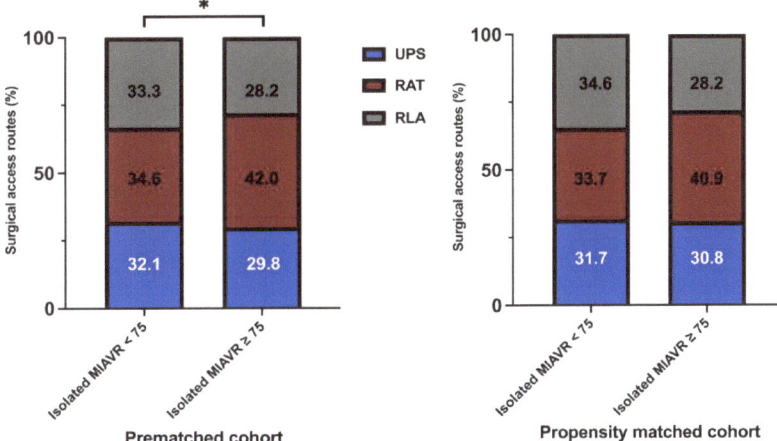

Figure 4. Distribution of surgical access routes within each treatment group. Abbreviations: UPS, upper partial sternotomy; RAT, right anterolateral thoracotomy; RLA, right lateral thoracotomy. Note: * $p < 0.05$ between groups. Note: As a consequence of the process of mathematical rounding, wherein percentages are rounded up or down to the nearest tenth decimal place, minute deviations of up to 0.1% from the absolute value of 100% can potentially manifest.

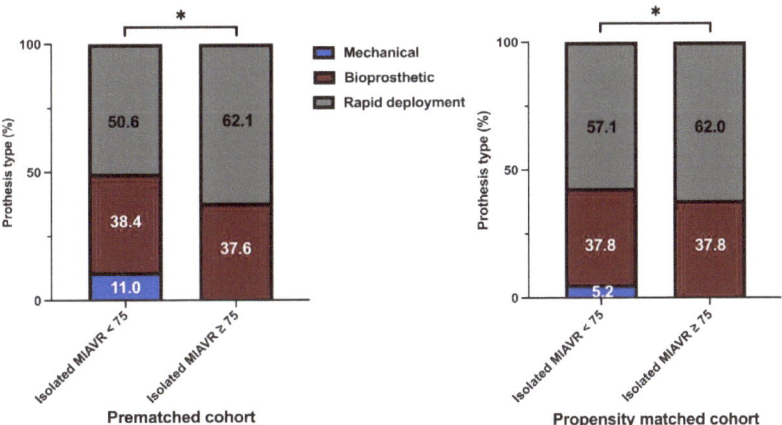

Figure 5. Distribution of aortic prosthesis type implanted within each treatment group. Note: * $p < 0.05$ between groups. As a consequence of the process of mathematical rounding, wherein percentages are rounded up or down to the nearest tenth decimal place, minute deviations of up to 0.1% from the absolute value of 100% can potentially manifest. The stacked column charts for the isolated MIAVR $\geq$75 cohort in both prematched and matched groups exclude the extremely small proportion (0.3% or 0.2% respectively) of mechanical valve prostheses. A graphical representation in this scale of this small quantity is not meaningful.

The primary postoperative ventilation time was shorter in the <75 group than in the $\geq$75 group ($p = 0.04$). Transfusion of packed red blood cells (PRBC) was performed less frequently in the <75 group than in the $\geq$75 group. Postoperative acute kidney injury (AKI) occurred more frequently in the $\geq$75 group (9.9%) than in the <75 group (4.9%; $p \leq 0.001$). When classified by grade, AKI grade II or III occurred more frequently in the $\geq$75 group (7.3%) than in the <75 group (3.8%; $p = 0.01$). Patients in the $\geq$75 group were significantly more likely to develop postoperative delirium than patients in the <75 group. Postoperative new-onset atrial fibrillation (NOAF) was significantly more common in the ≥75 group than in the <75 group. However, there were no significant differences in the 30-day mortality rate (1.5% vs. 1.8%; p = 0.82) or incidence of postoperative major adverse cardio-cerebral (MACCE) events, such as stroke (2.2% vs. 2.1%; $p \geq 0.99$), transient ischemic attack (0.9% vs. 0.8%; $p \geq 0.99$) and perioperative myocardial infarction (MI), between groups (Table 5).

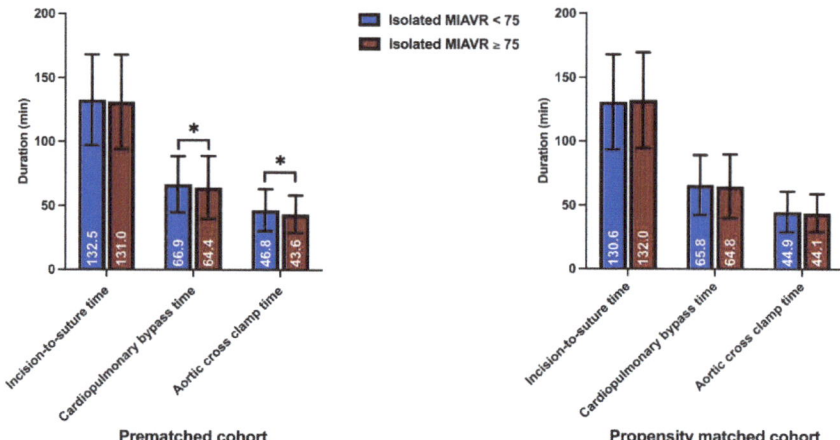

Figure 6. Surgical section times. Note: * p < 0.05 between groups.

Table 5. Postoperative morbidity and mortality.

	Pre-Matched Cohort			Propensity-Score-Matched Cohort		
	Isolated MIAVR < 75 (n = 956)	Isolated MIAVR ≥ 75 (n = 383)	p	Isolated MIAVR < 75 (n = 347)	Isolated MIAVR ≥ 75 (n = 347)	p
Ventilation time (hours)						
- ≤12, n (%)	869 (91.0)	333 (87.2)		110 (31.7)	107 (30.8)	
- ≤24, n (%)	57 (6.0)	33 (8.6)	0.04 *	117 (33.7)	142 (40.9)	0.10
- >24, n (%)	29 (3.0)	16 (4.2)		120 (34.6)	98 (28.2)	
Respiratory failure [†], n (%)	41 (4.3)	19 (5.0)	0.56	19 (5.5)	17 (4.9)	0.86
ICU stay (days), mean ± SD	2.1 ± 2.8	2.1 ± 2.1	0.17	2.4 ± 3.6	2.1 ± 1.9	0.57
Hospital stay (days), mean ± SD	9.9 ± 6.4	10.5 ± 5.0	≤0.001 **	11.0 ± 8.0	10.5 ± 5.0	0.11
Transfusion (PRBC), mean ± SD	0.7 ± 2.3	0.8 ± 3.6	0.02 *	0.9 ± 2.2	0.8 ± 3.7	0.16
AKI, n (%)	47 (4.9)	38 (9.9)	≤0.001 **	31 (9.0)	32 (9.2)	≥0.99
AKI grade II or III, n (%)	36 (3.8)	28 (7.3)	0.01 *	26 (7.5)	24 (6.9)	0.83
CVVH, n (%)	14 (1.5)	11 (2.9)	0.12	10 (2.9)	10 (2.9)	≥0.99
Conversion to sternotomy, n (%)	23 (2.4)	12 (3.1)	0.45	7 (2.0)	11 (3.2)	0.48
Rethoracotomy, n (%)	72 (7.5)	27 (7.1)	0.82	33 (9.5)	22 (6.4)	0.16
Impaired wound healing, n (%)	81 (8.5)	25 (6.5)	0.26	34 (9.8)	24 (6.9)	0.22
Postoperative delirium, n (%)	139 (14.6)	104 (27.2)	≤0.001 **	66 (19.1)	93 (26.9)	0.02 *
Ischemic stroke, n	21 (2.2)	8 (2.1)	≥0.99	9 (2.6)	5 (1.4)	0.06
TIA, n (%)	9 (0.9)	3 (0.8)	≥0.99	5 (1.4)	3 (0.9)	0.73
PPM implantation, n (%)	61 (6.4)	27 (7.1)	0.33	30 (8.7)	25 (7.2)	0.68
NOAF, n (%)	117 (12.3)	70 (18.3)	≤0.01 *	39 (11.3)	65 (18.8)	≤0.01 *
Myocardial infarction, n (%)	10 (1.0)	0 (0.0)	0.33	4 (1.2)	0 (0.0)	0.12
30-day mortality, n (%)	14 (1.5)	13 (3.4)	0.82	4 (1.2)	5 (1.4)	0.90

Note: Bold and italic values indicate statistical significance: *, $p \leq 0.05$; **, $p \leq 0.01$; [†], defined as primary postoperative ventilation time ≥72 h, reintubation and tracheotomy. Abbreviations: MIAVR, minimally invasive aortic valve replacement; AKI, acute kidney injury; CVVH, consecutive renal failure needing continuous venovenous hemofiltration; ICU, intensive care unit; PRBC, packed red blood cells; TIA, transient ischemic attack; NOAF, new-onset atrial fibrillation; PPM, permanent pacemaker.

The echocardiographic data obtained at discharge showed optimal prosthesis function in all patients. The transaortic peak and mean pressure were reduced significantly and did not differ between groups. Paravalvular regurgitation occurred at a similar frequency in both groups (Table 6).

Table 6. Echocardiographic data (on admission and at discharge).

	Pre-Matched Cohort			Propensity-Score-Matched Cohort		
	Isolated MIAVR < 75 (n = 956)	Isolated MIAVR ≥ 75 (n = 383)	p	Isolated MIAVR < 75 (n = 347)	Isolated MIAVR ≥ 75 (n = 347)	p
Preoperative AVA (cm^2), mean ± SD	0.7 ± 0.2	0.7 ± 0.2	0.34	0.7 ± 0.2	0.7 ± 0.1	0.89
Preoperative P$_{max}$ (mmHg), mean ± SD	78.4 ± 26.1	75.0 (21.8)	***0.01 ***	77.3 ± 32.3	73.8 ± 20.4	0.15
Preoperative P$_{mean}$ (mmHg), mean ± SD	47.6 ± 14.6	46.0 ± 15.0	***0.01 ***	46.7 ± 14.9	45.2 ± 14.1	0.12
Postoperative P$_{max}$ (mmHg), mean ± SD	24.8 ± 8.1	24.5 ± 7.9	0.70	11.0 ± 8.0	10.5 ± 5.0	0.11
Postoperative P$_{mean}$ (mmHg), mean ± SD	14.1 ± 4.6	14.0 ± 4.6	0.76	14.0 ± 4.7	14.1 ± 4.7	0.98
Paravalvular AR, n (%)	31 (3.3)	10 (2.6)	0.55	11 (3.2)	10 (2.9)	≥0.99
Paravalvular AR ≥ II, n (%)	13 (1.4)	4 (1.1)	0.30	2 (0.6)	4 (1.2)	0.68

Note: Bold and italic values indicate statistical significance: *, $p \leq 0.05$. Abbreviations: MIAVR, minimally invasive aortic valve replacement; AVA, aortic valve area; P$_{max}$, peak aortic valve gradient; P$_{mean}$, mean aortic valve gradient; AR, aortic regurgitation.

3.3. Outcomes of Propensity-Score-Matched Patients

After propensity score matching, we obtained 694 patients (347 pairs) for the matched analysis. Consistent with the unadjusted analysis, mechanical valves were more frequently implanted in the propensity-matched <75 group than in the ≥75 group (Figure 5).

Other procedural and intraoperative variables did not differ significantly between propensity-matched groups. The detailed procedural and intraoperative data are shown in Tables 2 and 3. The rates of postoperative delirium (26.9% vs. 19.1%; p = 0.02) and NOAF (18.8 vs. 11.3; p = 0.01) were significantly higher in the propensity-matched ≥75 group than in the <75 group. However, the 30-day mortality, MACCE and composite major morbidity did not differ significantly between groups (Table 5). Echocardiographic data did not differ significantly between groups (Table 6). The graphical overview of the postoperative outcomes of propensity-matched groups is shown in Figure 7.

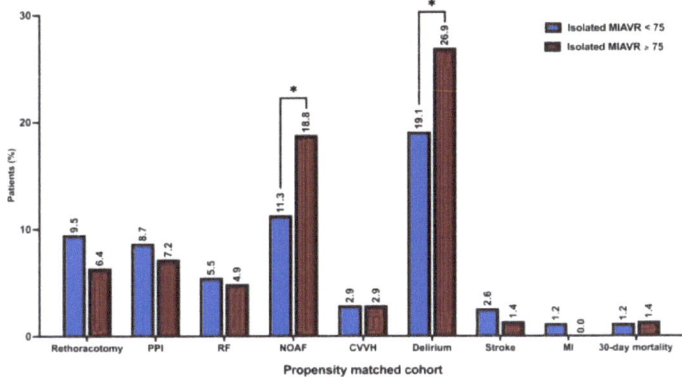

Figure 7. Postoperative outcomes. Abbreviations: PPI, permanent pacemaker implantation; RF, respiratory failure; NOAF, new-onset atrial fibrillation; CVVH, continuous veno-venous hemofiltration; MI, myocardial infarction. Note: * p < 0.05 between groups.

4. Discussion

As the indication for catheter-based valve procedures has expanded from high-risk patients to increasingly intermediate- and low-risk patients, TAVI has fundamentally changed the treatment regimen for patients with aortic valve stenosis. This trend found its way into the 2021 ESC/EACTS guidelines, postulating an age threshold favoring TAVI in patients ≥75 years [1]. The 2020 ACC/AHA guidelines go even further, discussing an age threshold of 65 years [8].

Nevertheless, the results from the OBSERVANT trial and the GARY registry have recently shown that TAVI patients have worse survival and a higher risk of serious cardiac and cerebrovascular events at five years compared with SAVR [9,10]. Additionally, a recent meta-analysis by Barili and colleagues demonstrated that "TAVI becomes a risk-factor for all-cause mortality and the composite endpoint [of death or stroke] after 24 months and for rehospitalization after 6 months" [11]. However, the ESC/EACTS guidelines also contain an interesting statement—but only for the curious readers, whose interest goes beyond the tables included. It is said therein that an age cut-off might be problematic, and in the individual case, the patient's life expectancy and the assumed durability of the catheter heart valve must be weighed up [1].

Considering this statement, taken together with the data published by Barili and colleagues—knowing that the average life expectancy of women and men aged 75 in Europe is 12–15 and 10–12 years, respectively—one could argue that every patient who has a life expectancy exceeding 5 years should undergo surgery, independent of their numeric age [11,12].

These considerations overshadow the unilateral support for the guideline recommendation in favor of TAVI for patients ≥ 75 years or even 65 years. Most previous randomized controlled clinical trials have compared SAVR with TAVI, usually focusing on the assessed surgical risk. Neither of these studies evaluated outcomes based on age, except for the NOTION trial. Furthermore, no distinction was made between conventional and minimally invasive access methods. We believe this is a methodical shortcoming. Recently, Wilbring et al., from our working group, demonstrated in a large-scale propensity-matched trial that transaxillary MIAVR was at least as safe as conventional SAVR using sternotomy but had the advantages of shorter hospital stay, shorter ventilation times, fewer transfusions, shorter ICU stay and bisected expected vs. observed mortality [13]. These results—with awareness of the increasing patient demand for less trauma, less pain and faster recovery—cast a slur on sticking to the classic sternotomy approach. It is quite understandable that in the age of TAVI, no patient is really convinced of sternotomy. MIAVR can be a strong argument in the discussion with a patient, as it is in Heart Team's discussion. At our institution, we advocate an institutionalized MIAVR strategy. This resulted in a 97.2% MIAVR rate in isolated aortic valve surgery, abolishing sternotomy almost completely and helping increase the number of SAVR procedures by around 20% from 2014 to 2022 [14].

Therefore, this study only reports the outcomes of isolated MIAVR in 1339 patients divided into two age-based groups according to a 75-year cut-off, followed by a propensity-score-matching analysis of 694 patients (347 pairs). No statistically significant difference in 30-day mortality was detected with either unadjusted or propensity-score-matched data. However, the mortality risk stratification scores for 30-day mortality (EuroSCORE II and STS-PROM) were significantly higher in the ≥75 group than in the <75 group. Similarly, no significant differences were found in perioperative stroke, transient ischemic attack (TIA) or MI incidence. The surgical arm of the NOTION trial, with a mean EuroSCORE II of 2.0% and mean age of 79 years in the full cohort, reported a notably higher 30-day mortality rate (3.7%) and perioperative stroke incidence (3.0%) than our patients aged ≥ 75 years. It should be noted that the recording of perioperative stroke events in our study was completely independent of clinical symptom severity or graduation according to the modified Rankin scale. Therefore, stroke event was assessed in case of any neurological deficits, and the corresponding computed tomographic data were correlated.

Previous studies identified older age as an independent NOAF predictor after SAVR [15–17]. Consistent with the results of these studies, postoperative NOAF occurred significantly more frequently in patients ≥ 75 years of age in our study. Advanced age is also an independent risk factor for postoperative delirium after cardiac surgery [18]. In accordance with these findings, the incidence of postoperative delirium was higher in the ≥ 75 group than in the <75 group in both the pre-matched and propensity-matched analyses.

In the pre-matched analysis, longer CPBT and ACCT were observed in the <75 group than in the ≥ 75 group. The cause of this observation remains unclear in the present data, especially since it was not reproduced in the propensity-score-matched analysis. The need for blood transfusion was significantly higher in the ≥ 75 group than in the <75 group in the unadjusted analysis. One possible reason for this could be the higher incidence of anemia in older age [19]. However, this finding was not reproduced in the propensity-matched analysis. The higher AKI rate in the pre-matched ≥ 75 group than in the <75 group was also not reproduced in the propensity-matched cohort. The higher AKI rate in the unadjusted ≥ 75 group, most likely related to already decreased preoperative creatinine clearance, did not differ significantly between the propensity-matched groups.

5. Limitations

This study has inherent limitations. First and foremost, despite its large cohort, this was a single-center retrospective study with only short-term follow-up. Second, our propensity-score-matching model might not have incorporated unknown but potentially relevant risk factors and confounders. Another potential problem arises from the fact that matching parameters were selected primarily based on surgical feasibility in minimally invasive aortic valve replacement procedures, resulting in incomplete matching of baseline characteristics (arterial hypertension, carotid artery stenosis, preoperative permanent pacemaker and preoperative hemodialysis). Furthermore, these MIAVR results were achieved in a high-volume expert center and cannot be extrapolated to all patients.

6. Conclusions

The aim and perspective of the present study are founded in the belief that TAVI is a great therapy, which has profoundly changed the treatment of valvular heart disease. Nonetheless, the decision-making process for TAVI or SAVR must be based on evidence. While TAVI has gained recognition as an effective treatment for high-grade aortic valve stenosis, we question the evidence-based data supporting the recommended age limit of 75 years. The present European guidelines suggest that an age threshold of 75 years is a long-standing legitimate decision parameter, despite the lack of evidence for "75 years" [1,20,21]. In our study, we aimed to compare the short-term outcomes of MIAVR in two age groups, specifically those below and above 75 years, rather than comparisons with a cohort of patients who underwent TAVI. The focus was to investigate whether patients above 75 years of age experienced any disadvantages in terms of short-term outcomes compared to the younger group. Our study data clearly indicate that this was not the case. Therefore, in addition to presenting our study findings, we aim to provoke a reconsideration of this somewhat arbitrary age limit. In addition, this study may help improve the decision-making process for or against SAVR.

A further aspect is that it was shown by means of hard endpoints, such as survival and stroke, that MIAVR is at least not inferior to sternotomy. Furthermore, minimally invasive techniques unarguably find wider patient acceptance because they meet the demand for less trauma, less pain and better cosmesis. In counterpoint to TAVI, it is imperative to question the following thesis: given the well-documented advantages offered by modern minimally invasive techniques for aortic valve replacement compared with sternotomy, what justifies the hesitation to firmly establish minimally invasive aortic valve replacement (MIAVR) as the prevailing standard?

Overall, we hope to encourage the advancement of cardiac surgery and the development of minimally invasive surgical approaches as suitable therapeutic options for older patients. Although our study's observation period was short, the results suggest that the minimally invasive approach is justified for patients above 75 years of age as well.

Author Contributions: Conceptualization, K.M., K.A., U.K. and S.A.; methodology, M.W., S.A. and A.T.-W.; software, A.P. and A.T.-W.; validation, M.W.; formal analysis, A.T.-W.; investigations, P.J. and A.T.-W.; data curation, P.J., A.P. and A.T.-W.; writing—original draft preparation, A.T.-W.; writing—review and editing, M.W., U.K. and S.A.; visualization, A.P. and A.T.-W.; supervision, S.A.; project administration, K.M. All authors have read and agreed to the published version of the manuscript.

Funding: This research received no external funding.

Institutional Review Board Statement: The study was conducted in accordance with the Declaration of Helsinki and approved by The Ethics Committee at the Technical University of Dresden (protocol code EK-25006222016 and EK-298092012).

Informed Consent Statement: Informed consent was obtained from all subjects involved in the study.

Data Availability Statement: The data presented in this study are available upon request from the corresponding author. The data are not publicly available due to ethical regulations.

Conflicts of Interest: The authors declare no conflict of interest.

References

1. Vahanian, A.; Beyersdorf, F.; Praz, F.; Milojevic, M.; Baldus, S.; Bauersachs, J.; Capodanno, D.; Conradi, L.; De Bonis, M.; De Paulis, R.; et al. 2021 ESC/EACTS guidelines for the management of valvular heart disease: Developed by the Task Force for the management of valvular heart disease of the European Society of Cardiology (ESC) and the European Association for Cardio-Thoracic Surgery (EACTS). *Rev. Esp. Cardiol.* **2022**, *75*, 524. [CrossRef] [PubMed]
2. Leon, M.B.; Smith, C.R.; Mack, M.; Miller, D.C.; Moses, J.W.; Svensson, L.G.; Tuzcu, E.M.; Webb, J.G.; Fontana, G.P.; Makkar, R.R.; et al. Transcatheter aortic-valve implantation for aortic stenosis in patients who cannot undergo surgery. *N. Engl. J. Med.* **2010**, *363*, 1597–1607. [CrossRef] [PubMed]
3. Leon, M.B.; Smith, C.R.; Mack, M.J.; Makkar, R.R.; Svensson, L.G.; Kodali, S.K.; Thourani, V.H.; Tuzcu, E.M.; Miller, D.C.; Herrmann, H.C.; et al. Transcatheter or surgical aortic-valve replacement in intermediate-risk patients. *N. Engl. J. Med.* **2016**, *374*, 1609–1620. [CrossRef] [PubMed]
4. Mack, M.J.; Leon, M.B. Transcatheter aortic-valve replacement in low-risk patients. *N. Engl. J. Med.* **2019**, *381*, 684–685. [CrossRef] [PubMed]
5. Reardon, M.J.; Van Mieghem, N.M.; Popma, J.J. Surgical or transcatheter aortic-valve replacement. *N. Engl. J. Med.* **2017**, *377*, 197–198. [CrossRef] [PubMed]
6. Barker, C.M.; Reardon, M.J. The corevalve US pivotal trial. *Semin. Thorac. Cardiovasc. Surg.* **2014**, *26*, 179–186. [CrossRef] [PubMed]
7. Thyregod, H.G.; Steinbruchel, D.A.; Ihlemann, N.; Nissen, H.; Kjeldsen, B.J.; Petursson, P.; Chang, Y.; Franzen, O.W.; Engstrom, T.; Clemmensen, P.; et al. Transcatheter versus surgical aortic valve replacement in patients with severe aortic valve stenosis: 1-year results from the all-comers notion randomized clinical trial. *J. Am. Coll. Cardiol.* **2015**, *65*, 2184–2194. [CrossRef] [PubMed]
8. Otto, C.M.; Nishimura, R.A.; Bonow, R.O.; Carabello, B.A.; Erwin, J.P., 3rd; Gentile, F.; Jneid, H.; Krieger, E.V.; Mack, M.; McLeod, C.; et al. 2020 ACC/AHA guideline for the management of patients with valvular heart disease: A report of the American College of Cardiology/American Heart Association Joint Committee on clinical practice guidelines. *Circulation* **2021**, *143*, e72–e227. [CrossRef] [PubMed]
9. Barbanti, M.; Tamburino, C.; D'Errigo, P.; Biancari, F.; Ranucci, M.; Rosato, S.; Santoro, G.; Fusco, D.; Seccareccia, F.; OBSERVANT Research Group. Five-year outcomes of transfemoral transcatheter aortic valve replacement or surgical aortic valve replacement in a real world population. *Circ. Cardiovasc. Interv.* **2019**, *12*, e007825. [CrossRef] [PubMed]
10. Beyersdorf, F.; Bauer, T.; Freemantle, N.; Walther, T.; Frerker, C.; Herrmann, E.; Bleiziffer, S.; Mollmann, H.; Landwehr, S.; Ensminger, S.; et al. Five-year outcome in 18 010 patients from the German aortic valve registry. *Eur. J. Cardiothorac. Surg.* **2021**, *60*, 1139–1146. [CrossRef] [PubMed]
11. Barili, F.; Freemantle, N.; Musumeci, F.; Martin, B.; Anselmi, A.; Rinaldi, M.; Kaul, S.; Rodriguez-Roda, J.; Di Mauro, M.; Folliguet, T.; et al. Five-year outcomes in trials comparing transcatheter aortic valve implantation versus surgical aortic valve replacement: A pooled meta-analysis of reconstructed time-to-event data. *Eur. J. Cardiothorac. Surg.* **2022**, *61*, 977–987. [CrossRef] [PubMed]

12. Recent Trends in Life Expectancy at Older Ages: Update to 2014. Available online: https://assets.publishing.service.gov.uk/government/uploads/system/uploads/attachment_data/file/499252/Recent_trends_in_life_expectancy_at_older_ages_2014_update.pdf (accessed on 26 February 2023).
13. Wilbring, M.; Alexiou, K.; Schmidt, T.; Petrov, A.; Taghizadeh-Waghefi, A.; Charitos, E.; Matschke, K.; Arzt, S.; Kappert, U. Safety and efficacy of the transaxillary access for minimally invasive aortic valve surgery. *Medicina* **2023**, *59*, 160. [CrossRef] [PubMed]
14. Wilbring, M.; Arzt, S.; Alexiou, K.; Charitos, E.; Matschke, K.; Kappert, U. Clinical safety and efficacy of the transaxillary access route for minimally invasive aortic valve replacement. *Thorac. Cardiovasc. Surg.* **2023**, *71*, S1–S72. [CrossRef]
15. Mariscalco, G.; Biancari, F.; Zanobini, M.; Cottini, M.; Piffaretti, G.; Saccocci, M.; Banach, M.; Beghi, C.; Angelini, G.D. Bedside tool for predicting the risk of postoperative atrial fibrillation after cardiac surgery: The POAF score. *J. Am. Heart Assoc.* **2014**, *3*, e000752. [CrossRef] [PubMed]
16. Jorgensen, T.H.; Thygesen, J.B.; Thyregod, H.G.; Svendsen, J.H.; Sondergaard, L. New-onset atrial fibrillation after surgical aortic valve replacement and transcatheter aortic valve implantation: A concise review. *J. Invasive Cardiol.* **2015**, *27*, 41–47. [PubMed]
17. Axtell, A.L.; Moonsamy, P.; Melnitchouk, S.; Tolis, G.; Jassar, A.S.; D'Alessandro, D.A.; Villavicencio, M.A.; Cameron, D.E.; Sundt, T.M., 3rd. Preoperative predictors of new-onset prolonged atrial fibrillation after surgical aortic valve replacement. *J. Thorac. Cardiovasc. Surg.* **2020**, *159*, 1407–1414. [CrossRef] [PubMed]
18. Afonso, A.; Scurlock, C.; Reich, D.; Raikhelkar, J.; Hossain, S.; Bodian, C.; Krol, M.; Flynn, B. Predictive model for postoperative delirium in cardiac surgical patients. *Semin. Cardiothorac. Vasc. Anesth.* **2010**, *14*, 212–217. [CrossRef] [PubMed]
19. Bach, V.; Schruckmayer, G.; Sam, I.; Kemmler, G.; Stauder, R. Prevalence and possible causes of anemia in the elderly: A cross-sectional analysis of a large European university hospital cohort. *Clin. Interv. Aging* **2014**, *9*, 1187–1196. [CrossRef] [PubMed]
20. Cremer, J. Wie aus leitlinien leidlinien werden! *Zeitschrift für Herz-Thorax- und Gefäßchirurgie* **2021**, *35*, 253–254. [CrossRef]
21. Dayan, V.; Gomes, W.J. The new esc/eacts recommendations for transcatheter aortic valve implantation go too far. *Eur. Heart J.* **2022**, *43*, 2753–2755. [CrossRef] [PubMed]

Disclaimer/Publisher's Note: The statements, opinions and data contained in all publications are solely those of the individual author(s) and contributor(s) and not of MDPI and/or the editor(s). MDPI and/or the editor(s) disclaim responsibility for any injury to people or property resulting from any ideas, methods, instructions or products referred to in the content.

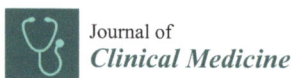 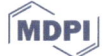

Article

Patient-Centred Outcomes after Totally Endoscopic Cardiac Surgery: One-Year Follow-Up

Jade Claessens [1,2,*,†], Pieter Goris [3], Alaaddin Yilmaz [2,†], Silke Van Genechten [2], Marithé Claes [3], Loren Packlé [2], Maud Pierson [3], Jeroen Vandenbrande [3], Abdullah Kaya [1,2] and Björn Stessel [1,3]

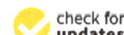

Citation: Claessens, J.; Goris, P.; Yilmaz, A.; Van Genechten, S.; Claes, M.; Packlé, L.; Pierson, M.; Vandenbrande, J.; Kaya, A.; Stessel, B. Patient-Centred Outcomes after Totally Endoscopic Cardiac Surgery: One-Year Follow-Up. *J. Clin. Med.* **2023**, *12*, 4406. https://doi.org/10.3390/jcm12134406

Academic Editors: Andrea Dell'Amore and Manuel Wilbring

Received: 5 May 2023
Revised: 31 May 2023
Accepted: 27 June 2023
Published: 30 June 2023

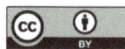

Copyright: © 2023 by the authors. Licensee MDPI, Basel, Switzerland. This article is an open access article distributed under the terms and conditions of the Creative Commons Attribution (CC BY) license (https://creativecommons.org/licenses/by/4.0/).

[1] Faculty of Medicine and Life Sciences, UHasselt—Hasselt University, Agoralaan, 3590 Diepenbeek, Belgium; abdullah.kaya@jessazh.be (A.K.); bjorn.stessel@jessazh.be (B.S.)
[2] Department of Cardiothoracic Surgery, Jessa Hospital, Stadsomvaart 11, 3500 Hasselt, Belgium; alaaddin.yilmaz@jessazh.be (A.Y.); silke.vangenechten@jessazh.be (S.V.G.); loren.packle@jessazh.be (L.P.)
[3] Department of Anesthesiology, Jessa Hospital, Stadsomvaart 11, 3500 Hasselt, Belgium; pieter.goris@jessazh.be (P.G.); marithe.claes@uhasselt.be (M.C.); piersonmaud@gmail.com (M.P.); jeroen.vandenbrande@jessazh.be (J.V.)
* Correspondence: jade.claessens@uhasselt.be; Tel.: +32-1133-7107
† These authors contributed equally to this work.

Abstract: Patient-centred outcomes have grown in popularity over recent years in surgical care research. These patient-centred outcomes can be measured through the health-related quality of life (HRQL) without professional interpretations. In May 2022, a study regarding patient-centred outcomes up to 90 days postoperatively was published. Fourteen days after surgery, the HRQL decreased and returned to baseline levels after 30 days. Next, the HRQL significantly improved 90 days postoperatively. However, this study only focuses on a short-term follow-up of the patients. Hence, this follow-up study aims to assess the HRQL one year after totally endoscopic cardiac surgery. At baseline, 14, 30, and 90 days, and one year after surgery, the HRQL was evaluated using a 36-item short form and 5-dimensional European QoL questionnaires (EQ-5D). Using the 36-Item short form questionnaire, a physical and mental component score is calculated. Over the period of one year, this physical and mental component score and the EQ-5D index value significantly improve. According to the visual analogue scale of the EQ-5D, patients score their health significantly higher one year postoperatively. In conclusion, after endoscopic cardiac surgery, the HRQL is significantly improved 90 days postoperatively and remains high one year afterward.

Keywords: quality of life; clinical outcomes; totally endoscopic cardiac surgery

1. Introduction

Research in the field of cardiac surgery predominantly focuses on reducing surgical trauma and improving the post-operative complications [1]. Recently, new totally endoscopic techniques were developed including totally endoscopic aortic valve replacement (TEAVR), endoscopic coronary artery bypass grafting (Endo-CABG), and mitral valve surgery through video-assisted thoracoscopic surgery (MVATS) [2–6]. Besides endoscopic AVR, transcatheter aortic valve implantation (TAVI) through the femoral artery has gained popularity and may be a viable alternative [7]. The aforementioned techniques are not yet state-of-the-art due to the technical difficulty and lack of clinical and patient-centred outcome data. Health-related quality of life (HRQL) is a measure of patient-centred outcomes that has gained importance in medical care. Through these outcome measures, the patient's health status can be determined without the interpretation of a physician, allowing for a better understanding of how surgery affects the patient's health [8]. The HRQL can be measured with questionnaires such as the short form 36 (SF-36) and the EuroQoL 5-dimension (EQ-5D). These questionnaires may meet the criteria for adequate surgical quality of recovery (QoR) measures [9]. There is a scarcity of prospective data on patient-centred outcomes, including HRQL and clinical results of these new totally endoscopic techniques. After our previously published study, which focused on patient-centred outcomes until 90 days after the surgery, the present study investigates the HRQL one year postoperatively [10]. In the previous study, the HRQL decreased over 14 days after surgery, then it returned to baseline levels at 30 days. After 90 days, the HRQL significantly improved. Our aforementioned study only focuses on a short-term follow-up of the patients. Hence, this follow-up study aims to assess the mid-term HRQL.

2. Materials and Methods

2.1. Study Design

This prospective longitudinal cohort study was authorized by Jessa Hospital's local ethics committee (registration number B243201836445), Belgium, and submitted for inclusion to clinicaltrials.gov (NCT03902717). The Declaration of Helsinki was followed in this trial, and all participants gave their written approval through an informed consent form.

Between November 2019 and October 2020, all patients undergoing totally endoscopic cardiac surgery (TECS), TAVI, or standard open CABG were eligible to participate. The TECS procedures included TEAVR, Endo-CABG, MVATS, and concomitant endoscopic treatments. An age below 18 years, involvement in another experiment, prior heart surgery, and conversion to sternotomy during the surgery were exclusion criteria. However, patients planned for a CABG through sternotomy were included. The HRQL was assessed through the SF-36 and EQ-5D questionnaires orally or over the phone. The different time points were baseline (before the surgery), 14, 30, and 90 days, and one year after the surgery. The study design was previously described [10].

2.2. Surgical Techniques

The description of the surgical techniques has been published before [2,6]. All procedures were performed using endoscopic ports (5 mm), a utility port (2–3 cm), and peripheral cardiopulmonary bypass (CPB).

2.3. Quality of Life

The two questionnaires used to assess the HRQL are the SF-36 and EQ-5D questionnaires [11,12]. The SF-36 includes eight domains, from which a physical and mental component score (PCS and MCS) can be calculated. The means and standard deviations from a reference population of people with ischemic heart disease in Belgium were used to standardize the eight SF-36 scales [13]. All values above or below 50 are above or below the average of the reference population. The higher the PCS and MCS score, the higher the HRQL of the patient. The eight domains of the SF-36 include physical functioning, role limitations due to physical health, pain, general health, role limitations due to emotional problems, energy/fatigue, emotional well-being, and social functioning. An index value for the EQ-5D is calculated based on a crosswalk value set (the general population of the Netherlands, since no data are available for Belgium). This index value is calculated from five dimensions: mobility, self-care, daily activities, pain/discomfort, and anxiety. Additionally, patients rate their current health on a scale from 0 to 100 in the EQ visual analogue scale (VAS).

2.4. Clinical Follow-Up

The clinical outcomes investigated in this trial were readmission, reoperation, major adverse cardiac and cerebrovascular events (MACCE, including cardiac death, stroke, myocardial infarction, and target lesion revascularization), and neurological complications (cerebrovascular accident (CVA) and transient ischemic attack (TIA)). Target lesion revascularization is defined as a reintervention in the target vessel for CABG, and in the valve procedures, a reintervention of the valve involved. Additional clinical outcomes included graft failure, paravalvular leakage, permanent pacemaker (PPM) implantation, pericarditis, and 30-day and one-year mortality. Pericarditis is defined as the presence of two of the following criteria: a pericardial friction rub, retrosternal chest pain, ECG changes (wide-spread concave ST-segment elevation and PR-segment depression), and/or pericardial effusion [14].

2.5. Statistical Analysis

The Shapiro–Wilk test was used to determine whether the data were normally distributed. Continuous variables were displayed as the median and interquartile range (IQR). Numbers and associated percentages provided the description of categorical variables. For non-parametric data, a Kruskal–Wallis test was used to compare the various surgical techniques, and a chi-square test was applied for categorical variables. The differences between the baseline and postoperative HRQL were examined using the Friedman and Wilcoxon signed-rank tests. A Kaplan–Meier estimated survival plot was created for the 30-day and one-year mortality. A p-value smaller than or equal to 0.05 was considered significant. All statistical analyses were performed using R: A language and environment for statistical computing (R Core Team (2021), R Foundation for Statistical Computing, Vienna, Austria).

3. Results

Enrolment and follow-up numbers are displayed in a STROBE (strengthening the reporting of observational studies in epidemiology) flow chart in Figure 1.

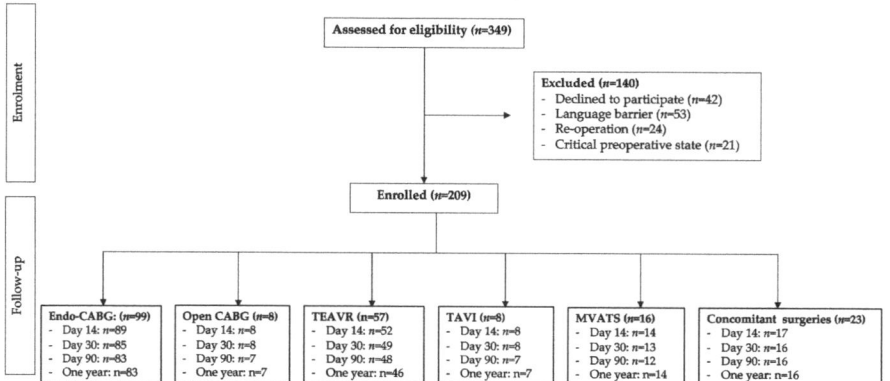

Figure 1. STROBE (strengthening the reporting of observational studies in epidemiology) flow chart of patient recruitment and follow-up. Endo-CABG: endoscopic coronary artery bypass grafting; TEAVR: totally endoscopic aortic valve replacement; TAVI: transcatheter aortic valve implantation; MVATS: mitral valve surgery through video-assisted thoracoscopic surgery.

3.1. Demographics

All subpopulations had similar outcomes except for the mean patient age in TEAVR versus TAVI ((73.0 (65.0–76.0) years versus 85.5 (77.8–87.8) years, $p < 0.001$) and the mean European system for cardiac operative risk evaluation (EuroSCORE) II in the open CABG group versus the Endo-CABG group, where the former was significantly higher (3.5 (1.9–4.6) versus 1.3 (0.9–2.2), $p = 0.021$). Demographics and medical history are described in Table 1 and in the previous manuscript [10].

Table 1. Demographics and medical history. Data are represented as n (%) and median (IQR).

	TECS (n = 193)	Endo-CABG (n = 99)	Open CABG (n = 8)	p-Value	TEAVR (n = 57)	TAVI (n = 8)	p-Value	MVATS (n = 16)	Concomitant (n = 23)
Age (years)	70.0 (62.0–77.0)	67.0 (61.5–73.5)	70.0 (68.0–75.5)	0.441	73.0 (65.0–76.0)	85.5 (77.8–87.8)	<0.001	72.5 (64.8–80.3)	75.0 (69.0–78.0)
BMI (kg/m^2)	26.9 (25.0–29.8)	26.7 (25.1–29.6)	27.8 (22.7–29.4)	0.859	27.0 (24.0–30.9)	26.0 (24.5–26.9)	0.259	26.1 (22.9–28.1)	27.6 (26.0–30.9)
EuroSCORE II (%)	1.6 (1.0–2.6)	1.3 (0.9–2.2)	3.5 (1.9–4.6)	0.021	1.4 (1.0–2.3)	-	-	2.3 (1.9–3.4)	2.7 (2.0–6.0)
Gender (male)	146 (75.6)	86 (86.8)	6 (75.0)	0.352	33 (57.9)	5 (62.5)	0.805	13 (81.3)	15 (65.2)
Smoking									
- Active	42 (21.8)	24 (24.2)	4 (50.0)	0.277	11 (19.3)	0 (0.0)	0.146	5 (31.3)	3 (13.0)
- Stopped	38 (19.7)	22 (22.2)	1 (12.5)		8 (14.0)	3 (37.5)		1 (6.3)	7 (30.4)
DiM									
- Type I	4 (2.1)	3 (3.0)	0 (0.0)	0.840	1 (1.75)	0 (0)	0.480	0 (0)	0 (0)
- Type II	44 (22.8)	29 (29.3)	2 (25.0)		6 (10.5)	2 (25.0)		3 (18.8)	7 (30.4)
AHT	130 (67.4)	70 (70.7)	7 (87.5)	0.309	35 (61.4)	5 (62.5)	0.952	7 (43.8)	20 (87.0)
Profession									
- Independent contractor	11 (5.7)	7 (7.1)	0 (0.0)	0.799	4 (7.0)	0 (0.0)	0.068	0 (0.0)	0 (0.0)
- Employed	18 (9.3)	9 (9.1)	1 (12.5)		6 (10.5)	0 (0.0)		2 (12.5)	1 (4.4)
- Volunteer	0 (0.0)	0 (0.0)	0 (0.0)		0 (0.0)	0 (0.0)		0 (0.0)	0 (0.0)
- Unemployed	5 (2.6)	2 (2.0)	0 (0.0)		0 (0.0)	0 (0.0)		2 (12.5)	1 (4.4)
- Incapacity of work	11 (5.7)	8 (8.1)	0 (0.0)		1 (1.8)	0 (0.0)		1 (6.3)	1 (4.4)
- Retired	148 (76.7)	73 (73.7)	7 (87.5)		46 (80.7)	8 (100.0)		11 (68.8)	20 (87.0)

Table 1. Cont.

		TECS (n = 193)	Endo-CABG (n = 99)	Open CABG (n = 8)	p-Value	TEAVR (n = 57)	TAVI (n = 8)	p-Value	MVATS (n = 16)	Concomitant (n = 23)
Education										
-	Elementary	20 (10.4)	12 (12.1)	1 (12.5)	0.696	5 (8.8)	3 (37.5)	0.067	1 (6.3)	2 (8.7)
-	Middle school	28 (14.5)	12 (12.1)	1 (12.5)		8 (14.0)	0 (0.0)		4 (25.0)	5 (21.7)
-	High school	91 (47.1)	44 (44.4)	2 (25)		30 (52.6)	4 (50.0)		6 (37.5)	22 (47.8)
-	Higher education	35 (18.1)	22 (22.2)	2 (25)		8 (14.0)	0 (0.0)		4 (25.0)	1 (4.4)
-	University	17 (8.8)	8 (8.1)	2 (25.0)		5 (8.8)	0 (0.0)		1 (6.3)	4 (17.4)
-	PhD	2 (1.0)	1 (1.0)	0 (0.0)		1 (1.8)	1 (12.5)		0 (0.0)	0 (0.0)

AHT: arterial hypertension; BMI: body mass index; DiM: diabetes mellitus; EuroSCORE II: European system for cardiac operative risk evaluation.

3.2. Health-Related Quality of Life

Totally endoscopic cardiac surgery: In the overall TECS cohort, the physical component score (PCS) of the SF-36 significantly changed after surgery ($p < 0.001$, Figure 2A). One year after the surgery, the PCS did not further improve compared to 90 days (90 days: 61.6 (55.1–65.6), one year: 61.8 (55.7–63.0), $p = 1$, Figure 2A). In contrast to the PCS, the MCS did not change significantly over the whole study period after TECS (Figure 2B). When comparing one year with 14, 30, and 90 days, the MCS did significantly improve (one year: 57.1 (52.3–61.4); 14 days: 51.0 (39.8–61.4), $p = 0.001$; 30 days: 53.7 (42.7–62.1), $p = 0.045$; and 90 days: 51.7 (39.6–61.0), $p = 0.001$) but compared to baseline values, there was no significant improvement after one year (56.5 (45.3–61.5), $p = 0.393$, Figure 2B).

Physical functioning, pain, general health, emotional well-being, and social functioning all improved over time. On the other hand, role limitations due to physical and mental health and the patient's energy/fatigue did not differ significantly over the five time points. Patients did not experience any role limitations due to mental health in any of the five time points. Additionally, an improvement was seen in role limitations due to physical health, pain, and social functioning between 90 days and one year (Figure S1).

In the overall TECS population, the EQ-5D questionnaire's index score significantly increased over time ($p < 0.001$). Compared to baseline values, a significant decline was observed after 14 days ($p < 0.001$), followed by a return to baseline values at 30 days and a significant increase at 90 days ($p = 0.015$), and the index score remained at these levels after one year (0.9 (0.8;1.0), $p < 0.001$, Figure 3A). Additionally, the EQ-VAS and index score results were similar to the evolution of the index score in the overall TECS populations (Figure 3B).

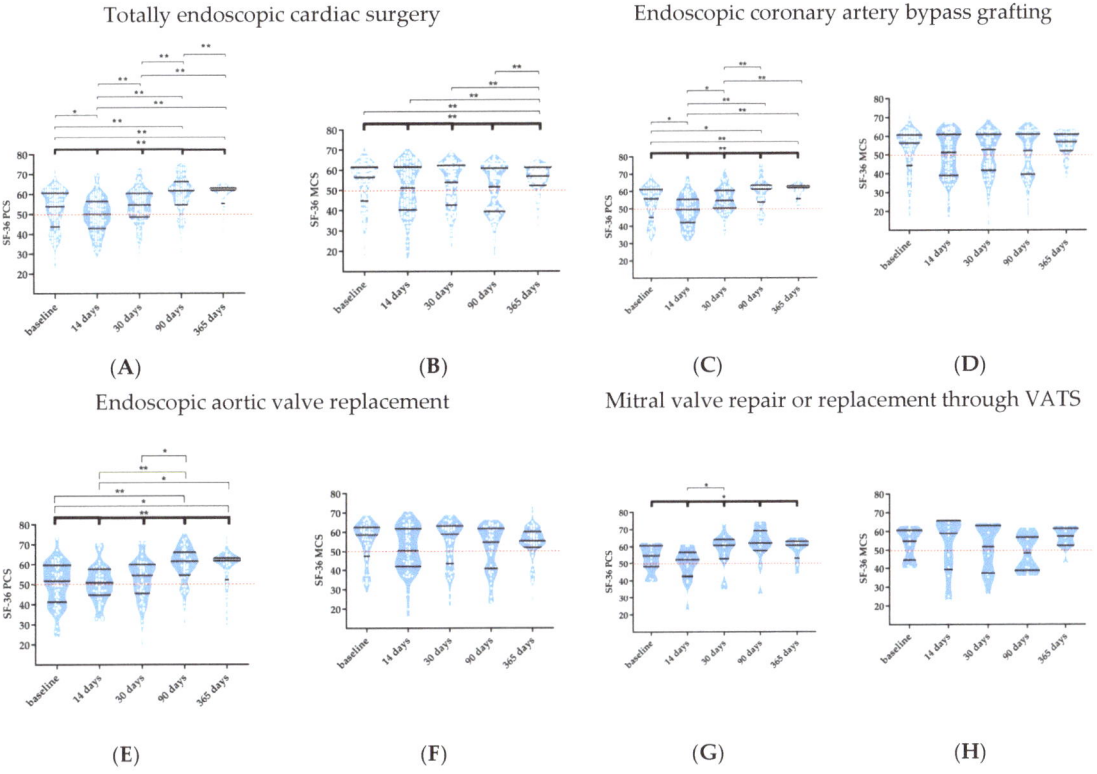

Figure 2. *Cont.*

Concomitant surgeries

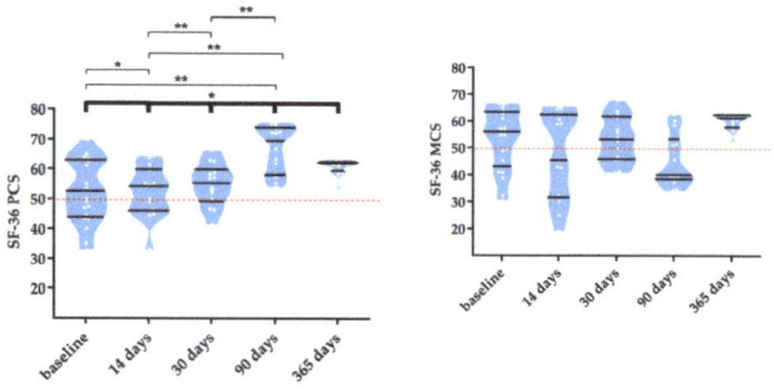

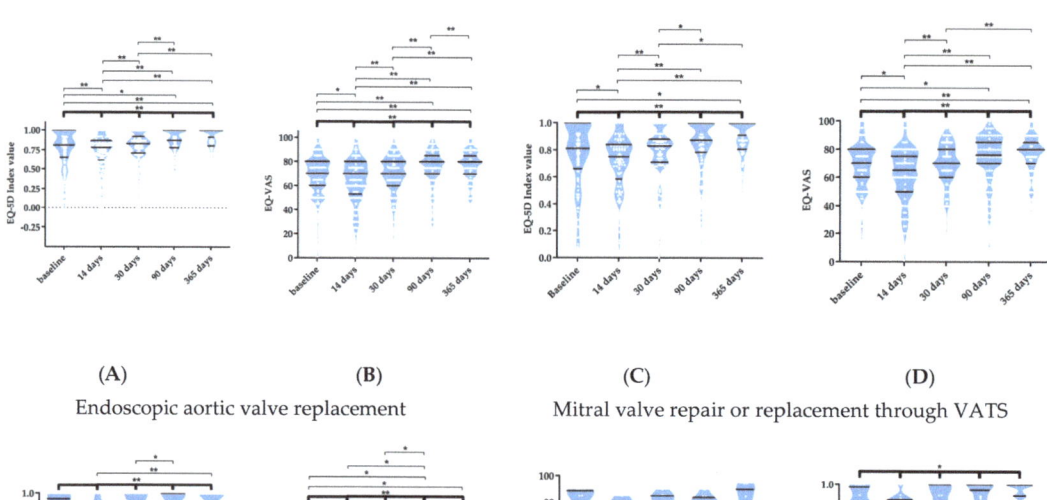

(I)   (J)

Figure 2. The physical and mental component scores (PCS and MCS) of the 36-item short form (SF-36) questionnaire after totally endoscopic cardiac surgery (**A**,**B**), endoscopic coronary artery bypass grafting (**C**,**D**), endoscopic aortic valve replacement (**E**,**F**), mitral valve repair or replacement through video-assisted thoracoscopic surgery (VATS) (**G**,**H**), and concomitant surgeries (**I**,**J**). Data are shown in truncated violin plots as medians and interquartile ranges. The reference line indicates the mean of a reference population (ischemic heart disease in Belgium, red line). The bold significance bar represents a Friedman analysis over the five time points. The other significance bars include post-hoc analyses using a pairwise Wilcoxon signed-rank test. Significance is marked as * $p < 0.05$ and ** $p < 0.001$.

Totally endoscopic cardiac surgery   Endoscopic coronary artery bypass grafting

(A)   (B)   (C)   (D)

Endoscopic aortic valve replacement   Mitral valve repair or replacement through VATS

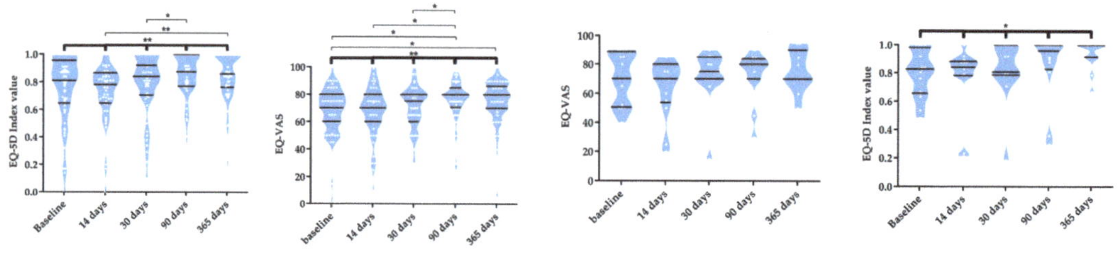

(E)   (F)   (G)   (H)

Figure 3. *Cont.*

Concomitant surgeries

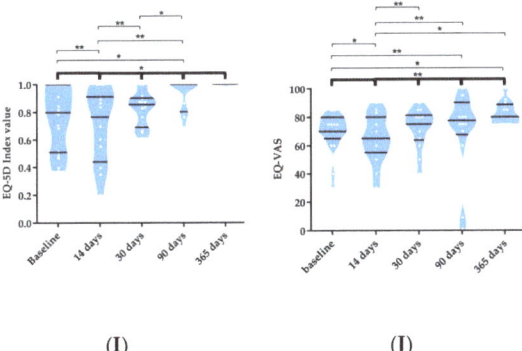

(I) (J)

Figure 3. The index value and visual analogue scale (VAS) of the European quality-of-life 5-dimensional questionnaire (EQ-5D) after totally endoscopic cardiac surgery (**A**,**B**), endoscopic coronary artery bypass grafting (**C**,**D**), endoscopic aortic valve replacement (**E**,**F**), mitral valve repair or replacement through video-assisted thoracoscopic surgery (**G**,**H**), and concomitant surgeries (**I**,**J**). Data are shown in truncated violin plots as medians and interquartile ranges. The bold significance bar represents a Friedman analysis over the five time points. The other significance bars include post-hoc analyses using a pairwise Wilcoxon signed-rank test. Significance is marked as * $p < 0.05$ and ** $p < 0.001$.

Coronary artery bypass grafting—The same significant improvements as the overall TECS population were seen in the PCS until one year after the surgery in the Endo-CABG patients ($p < 0.001$) with no further improvements between 90 days and one year ($p = 1$, Figure 2C). Following Endo-CABG, the MCS did not differ throughout the trial period (Figure 2D). Compared to open CABG, the PCS and MCS were not significantly different in the Endo-CABG group at different points in time ($p = 0.396$ and $p = 0.128$, respectively, Figure 4A,B).

In the Endo-CABG subpopulation, an improvement in physical functioning and role limitations due to physical health, pain, general health, and emotional well-being were observed over the five time points. The role limitations due to mental health and the patient's energy/fatigue did not differ significantly over the five time points. In contrast to the other domains, social functioning levels decreased (Figure S2).

Moreover, both the EQ-5D index value and VAS significantly improved over the whole study period ($p < 0.001$ and $p < 0.001$) in the Endo-CABG subpopulation (Figure 3C,D). After open CABG, only the VAS significantly improved ($p = 0.009$). No significant difference can be observed in the EQ-5D index value and VAS when comparing open CABG to Endo-CABG.

Aortic valve replacement—Similar to the overall TECS and Endo-CABG subpopulations, significant improvements in PCS were seen until one year after the surgery in TEAVR (Figure 2E) ($p < 0.001$), with no improvements between 90 days and one year.

When comparing TEAVR and TAVI, no significant difference in the PCS and MCS was seen ($p = 0.759$ and $p = 0.221$, respectively, Figure 4C,D).

TEAVR patients significantly improved in physical functioning, pain levels, and general health. The other domains of the SF-36 did not change over the different time points. Moreover, social functioning is the only domain significantly better in the TEAVR subpopulation compared to TAVI ($p = 0.031$, Figure S3). Additionally, the EQ-VAS and index score results were similar in the TEAVR and TAVI subpopulations.

Totally endoscopic mitral valve surgery—Patients who underwent a MVATS encountered similar significant improvements in PCS ($p = 0.028$) with no improvements between

90 days and one year. The MCS did not improve nor diminish over the whole study period. Additionally, emotional well-being was the only SF-36 domain that improved ($p = 0.030$). All other levels were high at all different time points (Figure S4).

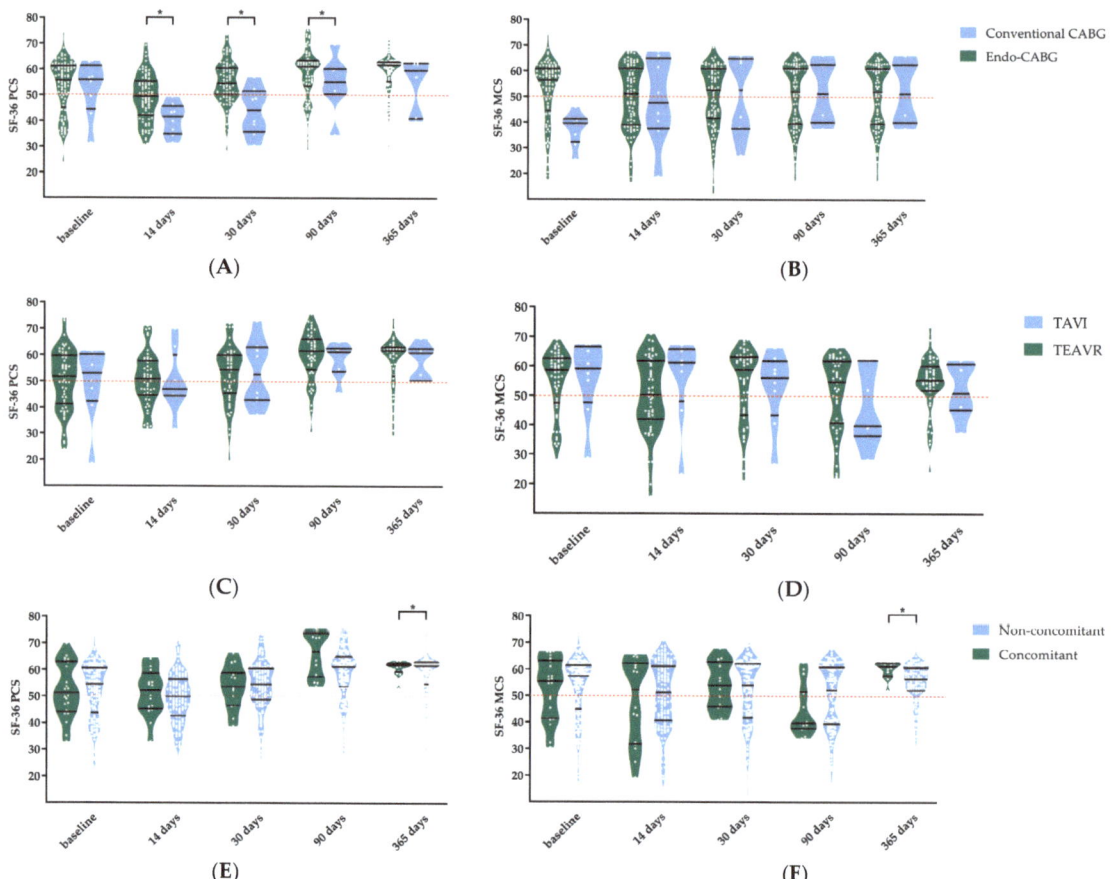

Figure 4. Comparison of the physical and mental component scores (PCS and MCS) of the short-form 36 (SF-36) questionnaire between endoscopic coronary artery bypass grafting (Endo-CABG) and open CABG (**A,B**), between totally endoscopic aortic valve replacement (TEAVR) and transcatheter aortic valve implantation (TAVI) (**C,D**), and between concomitant and non-concomitant (**E,F**). Data are shown in truncated violin plots as medians and interquartile ranges. The reference line indicates the mean of a reference population (ischemic heart disease in Belgium, red line). Significance is marked as * $p < 0.05$.

On the other hand, the EQ-5D index value significantly improved over the five time points ($p = 0.009$), while the VAS improvement was borderline not significant ($p = 0.059$).

Concomitant surgeries—As in all previously described populations, the same significant improvements in PCS were seen until one year after the concomitant surgeries ($p = 0.004$), with no further enhancements between 90 days and one year. Additionally, isolated TECS procedures compared to concomitant TECS showed no significant difference between the two for the PCS and MCS ($p = 0.273$ and $p = 0.716$, respectively, Figure 3E,F).

Furthermore, the EQ-5D index value and VAS significantly improved during the study after concomitant surgeries without any difference with single procedures.

3.3. Clinical Follow-Up

The clinical outcomes during the one-year follow-up period are presented in Table 2. In the overall TECS population, 28 (14.7%) patients were readmitted to the hospital 23.5 (15.8–53.8) days after the surgery, of which 8.9% were within 30 days. The reason for these readmissions included pericarditis, pleural effusion, heart failure, atrial fibrillation, hypotension, unstable angina, syncope, in-stent stenosis, and bradycardia. A reoperation was needed in three (1.6%) patients, two for a tamponade, and one Endo-CABG patient also required a TEAVR after 240 days. Furthermore, a MACCE occurred in 11 (5.8%) patients. These included five (2.6%) patients suffering a cardiac death, one (0.5%) patient with a myocardial infarction, and three patients with a stroke. Lastly, two patients needed a target lesion revascularisation.

Table 2. Clinical outcomes during the follow-up period of one year in endoscopic coronary artery bypass grafting (Endo-CABG), conventional coronary artery bypass grafting (CABG), totally endoscopic aortic valve replacement (TEAVR), transcatheter aortic valve implantation (TAVI), mitral valve repair or replacement through video-assisted thoracoscopic surgery (MVATS), and concomitant procedures.

	TECS (n = 193)	Endo-CABG (n = 99)	CABG (n = 8)	TEAVR (n = 57)	TAVI (n = 8)	MVATS (n = 16)	Concomitant (n = 23)
Readmission	28 (14.7)	18 (18.2)	0	7 (12.3)	0	2 (12.5)	2 (8.7)
Reoperation	3 (1.6)	1 (1.0)	0	1 (1.8)	0	1 (6.3)	0
MACCE	11 (5.8)	4 (4.0)	0	4 (7.0)	0	0	3 (13.0)
- Cardiac death	5 (2.6)	0	0	2 (3.5)	0	0	3 (13.0)
- MI	1 (0.5)	0	0	1 (1.8)	0	0	0
- Stroke	3 (1.6)	2 (2.0)	0	1 (1.8)	0	0	0
- TLR	2 (1.1)	2 (2.0)	0	0	0	0	0
Neurological							
- CVA	2 (1.0)	1 (1.0)	0	1 (1.8)	0	0	0
- TIA	2 (1.0)	2 (2.0)	0	0	0	0	0
Graft failure	1 (0.9)	1 (1.0)	0	-	-	-	0
Paravalvular leakage	0	-	-	0	3 (37.5)	0	-
PPM implantation	10 (5.2)	2 (2.0)	0	7 (12.3)	1 (12.5)	1 (6.3)	0
Pericarditis	25 (13.1)	16 (16.2)	0	7 (12.3)	0	1 (6.3)	1 (4.3)
Mortality	10 (5.2)	2 (2.0)	1 (12.5)	3 (5.3)	0	0	5 (21.7)
- In hospital	5 (2.6)	0	0	1 (1.8)	0	0	4 (17.4)
- 30-day	0	0	0	0	0	0	0
- Follow-up	5 (2.6)	2 (2.0)	1 (12.5)	2 (3.5)	0	0	1 (4.4)

CVA: cerebrovascular accident; MACCE: major adverse cardiac and cerebrovascular event; MI: myocardial infarction; PPM: permanent pacemaker implantation; TIA: transient ischemic attack; TLR: target lesion revascularization.

Paravalvular leakage was not diagnosed in the TEAVR, MVATS, or concomitant TECS subgroups. Within the TAVI subgroup, however, three patients developed a paravalvular leakage. A PPM implantation was performed in ten (5.2%) TECS patients. Pericarditis was diagnosed in 25 (13.1%) patients.

In total, 10 (5.2%) TECS patients died during the one-year follow-up period. Half of them were during the hospital stay, and the other half were between 30 days and one year. The estimated survival after one year for Endo-CABG, conventional CABG, TEAVR, and concomitant procedures was 97.7%, 87.5%, 94.0%, and 64.4%, respectively (Figure 5). Within the TAVI and MVATS subpopulations, none of the patients died.

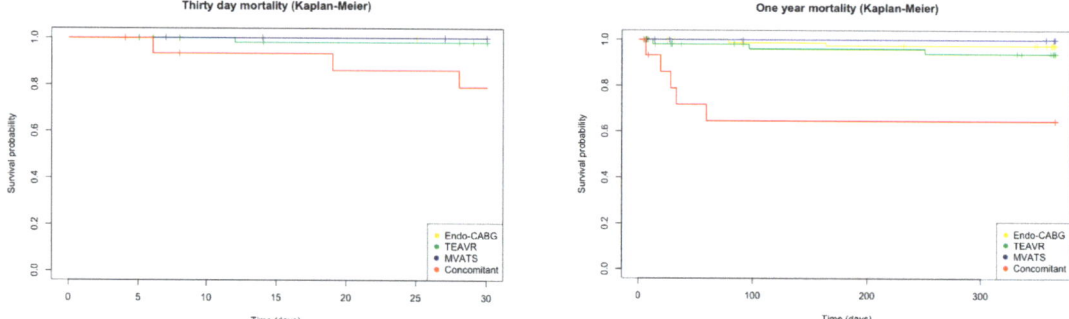

Figure 5. Estimated survival regarding the all-cause mortality (Kaplan–Meier) after 30 days and one year for endoscopic coronary artery bypass grafting (Endo-CABG), totally endoscopic aortic valve replacement (TEAVR), mitral valve repair or replacement through video-assisted thoracoscopic surgery (MVATS), and concomitant procedures.

4. Discussion

4.1. Overall HRQL

This trial investigated the quality of life after totally endoscopic cardiac surgery after a one-year follow-up. The SF-36 PCS and MCS did not change between 90 days and one year during the follow-up period in all investigated populations. Additionally, in the TECS population, the EQ-5D index value and VAS did not further improve after 90 days. According to the first part of this study, 14 days after TECS, there is a reduction in overall HRQL. Then, 30 days after the procedure, these levels revert to baseline, and at 90 days, they significantly improve. In the procedure-specific groups, comparable outcomes were seen. This indicates that the process of recovery takes place during the first three months after surgery. The initial recovery phase is followed by a plateau phase of a good HRQL during the year following the surgery.

Our results are consistent with the results of Moscarelli et al [15]. In their study, a difference in EQ-5D between minimally invasive and conventional valve surgery was seen at three months, while at one year, no difference was observed. When comparing our quality-of-life results after TECS with the results of Moscarelli et al. after MICS, TECS resulted in a higher index value (MICS: 0.6 ± 0.2 and TECS: 0.912 (0.8;1.0)) and VAS (MICS: 72.4 ± 12.6 and TECS: 80 (70;85)) at 90 days after surgery [15]. The faster immediate recovery and faster re-establishment of the HRQL compared to conventional sternotomy, as described by Moscarelli et al., was also observed by Nasso et al., who investigated minimally invasive mitral valve repair [15,16]. The swift recovery process resulting in a high HRQL at three to six months after surgery observed in these two studies and our study may explain the lack of further improvement between 90 days and one year. A systematic review of studies investigating the HRQL measured with the SF-36 and EQ-5D after minimally invasive cardiac surgery indicated that, while both minimally invasive and traditional cardiac surgery may benefit the patient, those receiving minimally invasive cardiac surgery may recover more rapidly [17].

4.2. Clinical Follow-Up

At one year of follow-up after TECS, the clinical outcomes were promising. After Endo-CABG, a MACCE was observed in only 4.0%. Two studies investigating conventional CABG reported a MACCE rate of 5.1% and 7.7% [18,19]. In contrast, we did not observe a MACCE in the conventional CABG subpopulation of this study. This finding can be explained by the small sample size ($n = 8$) of this subgroup. This explanation also applies to the TAVI subgroup of this study ($n = 8$), in which no MACCE was seen also. Other studies reported a MACCE rate of 12% and 18.2% after TAVI and a MACCE rate of 15.8% and 17.6% after conventional open AVR [20,21]. In this trial, 7.0% of TEAVR patients experienced a

MACCE. Moreover, the concomitant subpopulation had a higher occurrence of MACCE (13.0%) but aligned with the literature (11.5%) [22].

Furthermore, the readmission rate within 30 days was 8.9%, which is in line with the pooled 30-day readmission rate of 12.9% in the meta-analysis of Shawon et al. [23].

A PPM implantation was required in 5.2% of TECS patients. Especially after TEAVR, PPM implantation (12.3%) was higher compared to the literature (2–7%). The high PPM implantation rate observed in our study may be partially explained by a low threshold for pacemaker implantation at our hospital. In the literature, a PPM rate of 15.5% and 16.2% is reported after TAVI, which is still higher than in our TEAVR patients [20,21]. In this trial, the PPM rate of TAVI patients was also 12.5%. However, this depends on the type of valve prosthesis. In stented valves the PPM rate is significantly lower compared to sutureless valves. In this study, in 23.6% of patients, a sutureless valve was implanted.

The one-year mortality rate in the overall TECS population of this study was 5.2%, which is lower compared to other trials. After minimally invasive direct CABG, the reported mortality rate of 10.8% after a median follow-up of 11 months is five times higher than the observed mortality rate of 2.02% after Endo-CABG in our study [24]. Furthermore, after surgical AVR, the one-year mortality rate in other studies varies from 6.7% to 13.6%, compared to 5.3% in our study [20,25]. Regarding concomitant surgeries, the mortality rate (21.7%) observed in our study was higher than in other studies (8.4% and 11.0%). This observation may be partially due to the small sample size.

4.3. Limitations

In this study, the 30- and 90-day follow-up for most patients was during the COVID-19 pandemic, while the one-year follow-up was mainly afterwards. Presumably, the pandemic may have influenced our results regarding social and psychological functioning. For example, social functioning significantly improved after one year compared to 90 days. Several patients indicated that their social functioning was low due to the pandemic and not because of their health status.

Another limitation of this trial is the small sample size of the control groups (conventional CABG and TAVI). This is caused by the rapid switch to TECS in our centre. At the start of this trial, CABG was performed sporadically, and by the end of the trial, our centre became a 100% TECS centre. Regarding TAVI patients, the inclusion was more difficult due to the preoperative state of these patients. They were older, more fragile, and had more comorbidities, so they refused to participate in this trial more frequently. This created a huge selection bias between TEAVR and TAVI.

Lastly, the Hawthorne effect may always influence a trial with a questionnaire at multiple time points. Some patients may have reported higher HRQL due to the learning effect during the study period [26].

5. Conclusions

During the first three months after the surgery, the HRQL recovery process takes place. Following the initial phase of recovery, a plateau of a good HRQL is seen over the course of a year after surgery. The clinical follow-up during this period shows excellent morbidity and mortality rates. Our results indicate that implementation of TECS in the standard of care can have a positive effect on the HRQL and clinical outcomes after the surgery.

Supplementary Materials: The following supporting information can be downloaded at: https://www.mdpi.com/article/10.3390/jcm12134406/s1: Figure S1: Different domains of the Short Form 36 (SF-36) questionnaire after totally endoscopic cardiac surgery.; Figure S2: Different domains of the Short Form 36 (SF-36) questionnaire after totally endoscopic coronary artery bypass grafting; Figure S3: Different domains of the Short Form 36 (SF-36) questionnaire after totally endoscopic aortic valve replacement; Figure S4: Different domains of the Short Form 36 (SF-36) questionnaire after mitral valve repair or replacement through video assisted thoracoscopic surgery; Figure S5: Different domains of the Short Form 36 (SF-36) questionnaire after concomitant cardiac surgeries.

Author Contributions: B.S., S.V.G. and A.Y. conceived the study; J.C., M.C., M.P., L.P., P.G., J.V. and A.K. collected the data; J.C. performed the statistical analysis. All authors contributed to interpreting the results, and J.C. took the lead in writing the manuscript. All authors provided critical feedback. All authors have read and agreed to the published version of the manuscript.

Funding: This research received no external funding.

Institutional Review Board Statement: The study was conducted in accordance with the Declaration of Helsinki and approved by the Ethics Committee of Jessa Hospital, Belgium (registration number B243201836445) and registered on clinicaltrials.gov (NCT03902717).

Informed Consent Statement: Informed consent was obtained from all subjects involved in the study.

Data Availability Statement: The data underlying this article will be shared on reasonable request by the corresponding author.

Conflicts of Interest: The authors declare no conflict of interest.

References

1. Florence, Y.L.; Riccardo, G.A.; Bethany, T.; Tracy, K.; Gavin, J.M. Identifying research priorities in cardiac surgery: A report from the James Lind Alliance Priority Setting Partnership in adult heart surgery. *BMJ Open* **2020**, *10*, e038001. [CrossRef]
2. Yilmaz, A.; Robic, B.; Starinieri, P.; Polus, F.; Stinkens, R.; Stessel, B. A new viewpoint on endoscopic CABG: Technique description and clinical experience. *J. Cardiol.* **2020**, *75*, 614–620. [CrossRef]
3. Vola, M.; Fuzellier, J.F.; Chavent, B.; Duprey, A. First human totally endoscopic aortic valve replacement: An early report. *J. Thorac. Cardiovasc. Surg.* **2014**, *147*, 1091–1093. [CrossRef]
4. Mohr, F.W.; Falk, V.; Diegeler, A.; Walther, T.; van Son, J.A.; Autschbach, R. Minimally invasive port-access mitral valve surgery. *J. Thorac. Cardiovasc. Surg.* **1998**, *115*, 567–574. [CrossRef]
5. Jiang, Q.; Yu, T.; Huang, K.; Liu, L.; Zhang, X.; Hu, S. Feasibility, safety, and short-term outcome of totally thoracoscopic mitral valve procedure. *J. Cardiothorac. Surg.* **2018**, *13*, 133. [CrossRef]
6. Yilmaz, A.; Van Genechten, S.; Claessens, J.; Packlé, L.; Maessen, J.; Kaya, A. A totally endoscopic approach for aortic valve surgery. *Eur. J. Cardio-Thoracic Surg.* **2022**, *62*, ezac467. [CrossRef]
7. Webb, J.G.; Altwegg, L.; Masson, J.B.; Al Bugami, S.; Al Ali, A.; Boone, R.A. A new transcatheter aortic valve and percutaneous valve delivery system. *J. Am. Coll. Cardiol.* **2009**, *53*, 1855–1858. [CrossRef]
8. Desomer, A.; Van den Heede, K.; Triemstra Mattanja, T.; Paget, J.; De Boer, D.; Kohn, L.; Cleemput, I. *Use of Patient-Reported Outcome and Experience Measures in Patient Care and Policy*; KCE: Beaconsfield, Australia, 2018.
9. Tran, T.T.; Kaneva, P.; Mayo, N.E.; Fried, G.M.; Feldman, L.S. Short-stay surgery: What really happens after discharge? *Surgery* **2014**, *156*, 20–27. [CrossRef]
10. Claessens, J.; Yilmaz, A.; Mostien, T.; Van Genechten, S.; Claes, M.; Packlé, L.; Pierson, M.; Vandenbrande, J.; Kaya, A.; Stessel, B. 90-Day Patient-Centered Outcomes after Totally Endoscopic Cardiac Surgery: A Prospective Cohort Study. *J. Clin. Med.* **2022**, *11*, 2674. [CrossRef]
11. Razaval, D.; Gandek, B. Testing Dutch and French Translations of the SF-36 Health Survey among Blegian Angina Patient. *J. Clin. Epidemiol.* **1998**, *51*, 975–981. [CrossRef]
12. EuroQol. EQ-5D® is a Standardized Instrument for Use as a Measure of Health Outcome. 2019. Available online: https://euroqol.org (accessed on 29 April 2023).
13. Huber, A.; Oldridge, N.; Höfer, S. International SF-36 reference values in patients with ischemic heart disease. *Qual. Life Res.* **2016**, *25*, 2787–2798. [CrossRef]
14. Adler, Y.; Charron, P.; Imazio, M.; Badano, L.; Barón-Esquivias, G.; Bogaert, J.; Brucato, A.; Gueret, P.; Klingel, K.; Lionis, C.; et al. 2015 ESC Guidelines for the diagnosis and management of pericardial diseases: The Task Force for the Diagnosis and Management of Pericardial Diseases of the European Society of Cardiology (ESC)Endorsed by: The European Association for Cardio-Thoracic Surgery (EACTS). *Eur. Heart J.* **2015**, *36*, 2921–2964. [CrossRef]
15. Moscarelli, M.; Lorusso, R.; Abdullahi, Y.; Varone, E.; Marotta, M.; Solinas, M.; Casula, R.; Parlanti, A.; Speziale, G.; Fattouch, K.; et al. The Effect of Minimally Invasive Surgery and Sternotomy on Physical Activity and Quality of Life. *Heart Lung Circ.* **2021**, *30*, 882–887. [CrossRef]
16. Nasso, G.; Bonifazi, R.; Romano, V.; Bartolomucci, F.; Rosano, G.; Massari, F.; Fattouch, K.; Del Prete, G.; Riccioni, G.; Del Giglio, M.; et al. Three-year results of repaired Barlow mitral valves via right minithoracotomy versus median sternotomy in a randomized trial. *Cardiology* **2014**, *128*, 97–105. [CrossRef]
17. Claessens, J.; Rottiers, R.; Vandenbrande, J.; Gruyters, I.; Yilmaz, A.; Kaya, A.; Stessel, B. Quality of life in patients undergoing minimally invasive cardiac surgery: A systematic review. *Indian J. Thorac. Cardiovasc. Surg.* **2023**, *39*, 367–380. [CrossRef]

18. Caliskan, E.; Misfeld, M.; Sandner, S.; Böning, A.; Aramendi, J.; Salzberg, S.P.; Choi, Y.H.; Perrault, L.P.; Tekin, I.; Cuerpo, G.P.; et al. Clinical event rate in patients with and without left main disease undergoing isolated coronary artery bypass grafting: Results from the European DuraGraft Registry. *Eur. J. Cardio-Thoracic Surg.* **2022**, *62*, ezac403. [CrossRef]
19. Serruys, P.W.; Morice, M.-C.; Kappetein, A.P.; Colombo, A.; Holmes, D.R.; Mack, M.J.; Ståhle, E.; Feldman, T.E.; van den Brand, M.; Bass, E.J.; et al. Percutaneous Coronary Intervention versus Coronary-Artery Bypass Grafting for Severe Coronary Artery Disease. *N. Engl. J. Med.* **2009**, *360*, 961–972. [CrossRef]
20. Tamburino, C.; Barbanti, M.; D'Errigo, P.; Ranucci, M.; Onorati, F.; Covello, R.D.; Santini, F.; Rosato, S.; Santoro, G.; Fusco, D.; et al. 1-Year Outcomes After Transfemoral Transcatheter or Surgical Aortic Valve Replacement: Results From the Italian OBSERVANT Study. *J. Am. Coll. Cardiol.* **2015**, *66*, 804–812. [CrossRef]
21. Rosato, S.; Biancari, F.; D'Errigo, P.; Barbanti, M.; Tarantini, G.; Bedogni, F.; Ranucci, M.; Costa, G.; Juvonen, T.; Ussia, G.P.; et al. One-Year Outcomes after Surgical versus Transcatheter Aortic Valve Replacement with Newer Generation Devices. *J. Clin. Med.* **2021**, *10*, 3703. [CrossRef]
22. Alperi, A.; Mohammadi, S.; Campelo-Parada, F.; Munoz-Garcia, E.; Nombela-Franco, L.; Faroux, L.; Veiga, G.; Serra, V.; Fischer, Q.; Pascual, I.; et al. Transcatheter Versus Surgical Aortic Valve Replacement in Patients With Complex Coronary Artery Disease. *JACC Cardiovasc. Interv.* **2021**, *14*, 2490–2499. [CrossRef]
23. Shawon, M.S.R.; Odutola, M.; Falster, M.O.; Jorm, L.R. Patient and hospital factors associated with 30-day readmissions after coronary artery bypass graft (CABG) surgery: A systematic review and meta-analysis. *J. Cardiothorac. Surg.* **2021**, *16*, 172. [CrossRef] [PubMed]
24. Seo, D.H.; Kim, J.S.; Park, K.H.; Lim, C.; Chung, S.R.; Kim, D.J. Mid-Term Results of Minimally Invasive Direct Coronary Artery Bypass Grafting. *Korean J. Thorac. Cardiovasc. Surg.* **2018**, *51*, 8–14. [CrossRef]
25. Mohr, F.W.; Holzhey, D.; Möllmann, H.; Beckmann, A.; Veit, C.; Figulla, H.R.; Cremer, J.; Kuck, K.H.; Lange, R.; Zahn, R.; et al. The German Aortic Valve Registry: 1-year results from 13,680 patients with aortic valve disease. *Eur. J. Cardio-Thoracic Surg.* **2014**, *46*, 808–816. [CrossRef]
26. McCambridge, J.; Witton, J.; Elbourne, D.R. Systematic review of the Hawthorne effect: New concepts are needed to study research participation effects. *J. Clin. Epidemiol.* **2014**, *67*, 267–277. [CrossRef]

Disclaimer/Publisher's Note: The statements, opinions and data contained in all publications are solely those of the individual author(s) and contributor(s) and not of MDPI and/or the editor(s). MDPI and/or the editor(s) disclaim responsibility for any injury to people or property resulting from any ideas, methods, instructions or products referred to in the content.

MDPI AG
Grosspeteranlage 5
4052 Basel
Switzerland
Tel.: +41 61 683 77 34

Journal of Clinical Medicine Editorial Office
E-mail: jcm@mdpi.com
www.mdpi.com/journal/jcm

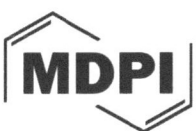

Disclaimer/Publisher's Note: The title and front matter of this reprint are at the discretion of the Guest Editor. The publisher is not responsible for their content or any associated concerns. The statements, opinions and data contained in all individual articles are solely those of the individual Editor and contributors and not of MDPI. MDPI disclaims responsibility for any injury to people or property resulting from any ideas, methods, instructions or products referred to in the content.

www.ingramcontent.com/pod-product-compliance
Lightning Source LLC
LaVergne TN
LVHW070002100526
838202LV00019B/2606